CHAKRAS FOR BEGINNERS

what the 7 main chakras are and how they

work; how to unlock them and balance them

with special techniques, to give off a great

positive energy and live a happy life

Table of Contents

INTRODUCTION

Chakras play a major role in those on a religious and holistic path. But what are they, exactly? Welcome to Beginners ' Chakras!

There are specific energy points inside the body. Such points are responsible for transmitting and receiving the power of life force in a spiral or circular motion. Such energy levels are commonly classified as chakras.

There are small chakras and large chakras. There are two lots of five small chakras between your hand's palm and shoulder, and also between your foot arch and the pelvis.

That leaves the seven big chakras most often addressed and the way to balance life and spiritual power!

Chakras respond very well to the vibration of sound and color. Each resonates in harmony with a certain color and a particular tone or note of music. You can restore the chakras to their original levels of health, strength, and clarity by visualizing the patterns and shades of each chakra. This is very important because the chakras are best tuned, light, open and spin smoothly–not too fast and not too slow. Let us address in more detail the seven major ones.

The chakra system is important to our mind, body and spirit's wellbeing. All in the world goes through a period. You will gain much inner knowledge and integrity by stimulating this cycle as you work toward a common goal.

Now that the fundamentals of chakras are understood, what they do and how they work, it's important to know that they don't just spin as they should. Things happen in life and everything from illness, shock, trauma and other causes cannot turn or shine as our chakras would. They need to be tuned and stimulated to keep them active. It is here that the art of chakra stimulation takes center stage.

Chakra Stimulation is an old technique used to increase spiritual awareness. Spiritual energy is the basis of every ability or power you currently have, and it is from the chakras that spiritual energy comes. It could be argued that our chakras are the most important thing to establish in our minds and bodies because they are a foundation for most other creatures.

You can use brain training to mimic the experiences of many years of profound spiritual development of yogis to improve the tuning and to activate the chakras to the maximum level of service. Just hearing these awesome bi-national beats and isochronic sounds, your brain is placed in such a position that operates on all your chakras at once or even grows and restores every single chakra, ensuring that they turn freely and shine brightly!

You will be shocked by the differences you experience as soon as your chakras are all aligned, tuned and stimulated! Like most meditation and deep alpha, theta and delta states, the purpose is to make sure the mind and brain are in the best brainwaves to achieve such amazing abilities.

CHAPTER ONE:
What Are Chakras?

But what are these chakras? Chakras can be called the Sanskrit wheel because of the movement of energy in the body. Let's extend the definition because we're talking about the body. The body usually has a composition of energy centers that can be called chakras because they look like spinning wheels. Such chakras are responsible for the flow of energy as it can flow from one place to another. Chakras are related to life's normality in that the tone, color, and light all interact with these energy centers correctly. Healing aims to balance chakras by correctly aligning them with a primary role of knowing nature as it is concerning the creation and human intent in existence.

The whole body has seven chakras strategically located. The first chakra also is known as the red chakra is found at the base of the spine and is also known as the chakra of the heart. Kundalini is another name for this chakra. The second chakra among the seven chakras is the spleen represented under the umbilical cord under the scar. Meditation leads to the awakening of the chakras, which means that without meditation the principle of manipulating chakras to achieve the desired balance can not be accomplished. The second chakra, however, is responsible for sexual ability and remorse is present once it is unbalanced.

The third chakra in the seven chakras is the solar plexus, which implies a place of feelings and it is what brings us power on the planet, as well as the yellow color, represents this chakra. The fourth chakra also is known as the chakra of the heart is expressed or shown in a sense of the soul's lack of compassion by the color green effects. The fifth chakra is depicted by the blue color and this emoticon, known as the throat, provides free speech during meditation. The sixth chakra until we sum it up the seventh chakras was the third eye and often emphasizes the forehead as a dominant in such energy factors, portrayed by the color indigo.

The seventh chakra that completes the deal on the seven chakras is the crown, represented by the purple color and intended to bind you to the higher realms. Chakras often manifest in the body as they absorb energy as they intensify with color, light, and sound. Prana is regarded as the divine power emanating from these chakras. Chakra centers swallow prana which causes them to vibrate where energy is created later. Once prana unites with the brain, we may assume that the primary goal of balancing chakras has been achieved.

Prana is the relation between the astral body and the living body. Meditation is the answer to many chakra questions. For example, how the energy is produced, how it moves, and what the benefits are. If you know the benefits of yoga asana, then you know that balancing chakras is another chance to call out the explosive energy that can bring one level of reality to another. This was rooted in astral flight and astral dimensions in most situations. The seven chakras ' vocabulary terms are Sahasrara, swadhishthana, Anahata, Manipura, aina, visudha and Muladhara. The purpose of these chakras is to represent the mental state concerning each energy center and translate it accordingly. Essentially, chakras of equilibrium are in that state only if their vibration can be attenuated at a given frequency. So when they are blocked, what are chakras. When one of the chakras or energy centers is blocked, it affects our physical health and therefore when people begin to get sick.

In other words, the energy centers are these aspects ' healing states. The energy centers that in this case are the chakras are properly represented in the forms of tantric texts in traditional Hinduism. Nevertheless, this theory has been related to prana in the modern world and can be circled back to the 18th century when a well-known scientist used animal magnetism as a treatment for a certain disease. The theory of chakras was closely related to this scientist's accomplishments, but on this phenomenon, there is still academic research.

Introduction to the Chakra System

The word chakra is a Sanskrit word that means wheel or circle and refers to the many energy centers that make up our bodies. These centers of energy are not visible to the human eye; however, some intuitive people can see one's chakras in the eye of their mind. There are hundreds of chakras in the human body, but concentrating on the 7 key chakras is only important. These central chakras are lined up to the top of the head from the base of the spine. That chakra is associated with a particular color and reflects certain parts of your physical, mental, and spiritual bodies.

• Your first chakra, also known as the root chakra, is at the base of your spine and vibrates at a red color level. The root chakra is your base chakra which helps you to meet basic needs including food, shelter, and water on earth. The chakra's physical aspect involves the blood and nervous systems, the spine, bladder, and organs of reproduction. A root chakra that is out of balance or blocked can cause depression, lack of trust, lethargy, inflammation, and rage; just to name a few.

• The second chakra, or sacral chakra, can be located just below the navel. This chakra vibrates at the rate of orange color and is related to our capacity to be imaginative, reproductive, and fertile (including being fertile with ideas, etc...). The sacral chakra functionally comprises the hair, lungs, mammary glands, and the reproductive system of women. A sacral chakra that is out of control or blocked can cause skin problems like rashes and acne, fertility issues, lack of creativity, violence, and emotional instability. It is this chakra that many people store certain emotions they have pushed down or not dealt with, so blocking this chakra is very simple.

• First, the 3rd chakra or solar plexus chakra below the ribs. This chakra vibrates at the yellow color level and is your source of internal energy and meaning for yourself. The liver, spleen, thyroid, and small intestine are the associated organs to the solar plexus. This chakra can cause digestive problems, diabetes, low self-esteem, low energy, and confusion out of balance.

• The connection between the lower 3 chakras (earth) and the upper 3 chakras (spiritual) is the fourth chakra or core chakra. The heart chakra is located directly in the middle of the chest and vibrates at the green color level (most people think the color is red, but this is the opposite green color on the color wheel). This chakra is all about esteem, self-love, and empathy, including the gland of the heart and breasts, endocrine, and thymus. Heart disease, allergies, chronic fatigue syndrome, envy, moodiness, and indifference can occur out of control.

• The fifth chakra or throat chakra lies in the stomach. The throat chakra vibrates at the color light blue level and is associated with voice, interaction, and self-expression. The chest, lungs, and ears are associated with organs. Hearing issues, asthma, sore throats, thyroid problems, pride, and confusion are complications that can result from an out-of-balance throat chakra.

• The 6th chakra or the sixth eye chakra (another name for this chakra is the brow chakra) is moving up to the middle of the forehead. This chakra vibrates at the Indigo color level and is connected to one's mind and intuitive abilities. The ears, lower head, and sinuses are connected to this chakra. This chakra can cause migraines, vision defects, sinus problems, dispersion and disorganization out of control, and an inability to trust your instincts.

• The last chakra is the seventh chakra also known as the crown chakra, located at the top of the head and linked to self-knowledge and spiritual consciousness. This chakra vibrates at the white color level which includes the full-color spectrum. The brain is the related organ to the chakra of the crown. Several symptoms can happen when depression is out of control, some cognitive and emotional conditions, dizziness, lack of contact with reality, and no other concern.

There are countless explanations why the chakras may become unbalanced or blocked and disrupt the flow of the entire system when one becomes clogged. Good care for your chakra system will help maximize your energy flow to make the most of your days. There are many basic strategies to keep the energy centers going out there, and I advise you to use whatever one feels right to you.

Chakras for Beginners

The human body has seven main sources of energy connected to the body's major organs and glands. Such energy centers are called chakras, and the Sanskrit word for wheel is chakra.

So, the human body's chakras are wheel-like spinning vortexes. To create a vacuum in the center and the process, they whirl in a circular motion, drawing everything they experience on their vibratory point.

Beginners searching for more information about chakras can find information stating that there are hundreds of chakras in the Buddhist scriptures, while there are nine chakras in the jains. Such knowledge should not confuse them as the most recognized chakras are the seven chakras.

These seven chakras are not marked in the human body, nor can they be identified or found. This is because these chakras are not part of the physical body but are all part of a human being's etheric or psychological body.

It can be said that this etheric body is split into different energy streams.

1. Muladhara or root chakra binding us to earth. Through concentrating on basic needs such as food, water, shelter, and sex, this chakra can be balanced.

3. Sacral chakra or Swadhisthana is found under the navel and is also known as a hard chakra. Fear, hate, rage, and aggression are its natural capacity. And all this can be balanced with one's doubts being embraced.

3. Solar plexus or Manipura is the fifth solar plexus chakra. There are two aspects of this chakra; doubt and confidence. Trust begins to develop here when doubt is transformed.

4. Heart Chakra or Anahata is the middle separating the seven chakras. This is the chakra responsible for building life's equilibrium. Our growth leads to a feeling of greater love for others and ourselves.

5. Throat chakra or Visshuddhi is the fifth chakra that allows you to become real in your life. When opened, this chakra's energy encourages you to communicate openly and allows you to truly express your viewpoint.

6. The body's third eye or Ajna is a very important chakra. It is located between the eyebrows and is known

as a person's third eye. When this third eye is opened one begins to develop self-awareness.

6. The Sahasrara or crown chakra is a bright white glow at the top of your head. This is the seventh chakra between body and mind, and the soul is linked to the other world through this chakra.

To beginners, this is enough knowledge to start gaining an understanding of the seven chakras. Just confusing you will be looking for additional details about the chakras. Beginners should learn to feel these chakras with the aid of individuals who have encountered these chakras.

When you begin to experience your chakras, you feel your body's energies flowing and you grow spiritually as lightness descends on you. Only if there are no obstructions and free-flowing energy makes the chakra travel do you feel this feeling.

CHAPTER TWO:

Aromatherapy to Balance the Chakras

Chakra is a Sanskrit word that means "water wheel." There are seven chakras in our bodies, each representing a different core of spiritual energy that transmits and receives power from and to Spirit (aka God, the Cosmos, etc.). Your physical and emotional wellbeing will be impaired if your chakra is out of control. Aromatherapy could be used as one way of balancing the chakras and helping you return to a calm, healthy and happy state of being. In this section , I will talk about the areas of the body that are regulated by each chakra, the features of a healthy and unbalanced chakra, the essential oils that can be used in aromatherapy to help balance the chakra and some examples of how these can be easily integrated into your daily life.

Red Essential Oils: Sandalwood, Peppermint, Cinnamon, Patchouli, Cloves The Root Chakra is the first chakra or foundation chakra. This binds our spirit to Mother Earth with our soul as well as our body. It's at the base of the backbone. The root chakra governs our survival and self-preservation impulses. The primordial chakra is linked to certain facets of our personalities such as feelings of safety and security as well as primary sexual desires. When the root chakra is balanced, we feel rooted, safe and full of life, busy, enthusiastic, capable of performing tasks, we feel strong, content and sexually healthy. Occasionally, however, due to unexpected circumstances such as the death of a loved one, the root chakra may be thrown out of control. These things have a way to turn our world inside out, and it's no wonder that our chakras and everything else will be thrown out of control. When the root chakra is out of control, one may feel scared, victimized, detached, and prone to explosions.

The Correspondence of the Sacral Chakra Color: Orange Essential Oils: Patchouli, Ylang Ylang, Sandalwood, Rose, Sage, Bergamot The Sacral Chakra is the second chakra and is found in the lower abdominal region just below the ring. Our emotions and sexuality are regulated by the sacral chakra. A person with a healthy sacral chakra enjoys great sexual energy and emotional awareness. When the sacral chakra is out of control, you can feel all the time either too emotional or vulnerable or at the other end of the spectrum, completely disconnected from others and emotionally unavailable. Sexual dysfunction, infidelity, and fear of intimacy are other indicators of an imbalance.

The Solar Plexus Chakra Color Correspondence: Yellow Essential Oils: Frankincense, Rose, Myrrh, Rosewood, Sandalwood, Chamomile, and Rosemary The Solar Plexus Chakra is the third chakra in the upper abdominal area, below the heart, above the belly button. Our sense of self, our self-esteem and the production of personal power are governed by the solar plexus chakra. They experience low self-esteem, fear of rejection, oversensitivity to criticism, fears of self-image and indecisiveness when the solar plexus chakra is out of control.

The Correspondence of the Heart Chakra Color: Green and Pink Essential Oils: Citrus Essential Oils (Lemon, Orange, Bergamot, etc.), Sandalwood, Ylang Ylang, Rose and Lavender The Heart Chakra is the fourth chakra in the heart. The chakra of the heart is all about healing and caring. Divorce or divorce, death of a loved one, emotional abuse, rejection or adultery are traumatic circumstances that can damage this chakra. We experience feelings of grief, anxiety, isolation when the heart chakra is out of control and we are unable to express love openly.

Blue Essential Oils: Peppermint, Spearmint, Chamomile, Bergamot and Basil The Throat Chakra is the fifth chakra and is found in the chest, throat, and ears. The throat chakra controls our ability to effectively communicate and to listen to and understand others. When the throat chakra is out of control, you may have trouble expressing yourself, repressing emotions, and having poor learning ability. Certain imbalance signs include repeated deception, anxiety, doubt, and confusion.

The Third Eye Chakra Color Correspondence: Indigo Essential Oils: Patchouli, Sandalwood, Clary Sage, Vetiver, Cypress and Juniper The Third Eye Chakra is the sixth chakra, found between the eyebrows on the forehead. Our capacity to use common sense, intellect, wisdom, dream perception, spirituality, and intuition is controlled by the third eye chakra. When the third eye chakra is out of control, there may be a lack of intelligence, common sense, forgetfulness, sleep problems, and uncertainty.

Correspondence from the Crown Chakra Color: White / Violet Essential Oils: Cedarwood, Frankincense, Jasmine, Lavender, Rose, and Sandalwood The Crown Chakra is the 7th chakra. The crown chakra, located at the top of the head, allows us to link with and interact with Spirit. You feel like you lack creativity and are spiritually detached when the crown chakra is out of control. You may become very materialistic, trapped in past pain, and preoccupied with the future. It may be your way to feel fulfilled to concentrate on material possessions.

I hope you've enjoyed reading about the chakras and their features, their correspondence of colors and essential oils that can be used to balance them. If you think any of your chakras are unbalanced, using aromatherapy along with relaxation can once again help you achieve equilibrium.

Here are some easy ways to help calm your chakras with aromatherapy.

•Take a bath or shower with products made from essential oils suited to the chakra.
• Use a tissue with a few drops of the ideal essential oil and breathe in a deep balance.
•During meditation, burn incense.
•Wear chakra color matching clothes or accessories when concentrating on maintaining balance and harmony.

Chakra Clearing - The Natural Way to Heal

Would you like more balance in your life? In your conditions, do you feel stuck? Looking for a safe way to heal your mind and body? Chakra meditation balance is the perfect tool because it operates with the strength of your own body.

The Chakra system is made up of seven stages corresponding to your body's different organs and structures. The word chakra comes from the ancient word Wheel in Sanskrit. The chakras are not in the physical body but the creative body. Each of us has seven major body chakras, shaped like a flower or wheel, with petals or spokes describing their structure. The energy in each chakra will influence your life's different circumstances. The chakras in your body absorb and process power, and just as you can be powered by energy, so it can obstruct you.

But, sometimes we all feel some kind of chakra imbalance, chakra healing aims to make all chakras work and spin smoothly and evenly, helping you balance your strength.

The seven key chakras are as follows:· The Root Chakra· The Sacred Chakra· The Chakra of the Solar Plexus· The Chakra of the Heart· The Chakra of the Throat· The Chakra of the Brow or the Chakra of the Third-Eye· The Chakra of the Crown Each chakra is associated with a color, a musical note and other things such as crystals or signs. Meditations with chakras are meant to cure and balance the body's strength.

This type of practice is a good way to balance your strength when you feel stressed and anxious as it revitalizes you from the inside out.

Knowing and controlling this energy will help you restore power and stability to your life, helping you to lead a happier and healthier life. Taking the time to balance your energy will help dissipate the energy of negativity and draw the things you so desire into your life and magnetic field.

Chakras, also known as Chi, are the source of your life force power or prana. The best way of thinking about your chakras is to picture them running up and down your spine like cogs or wheels, continually renewing your power. The chakras rotate clockwise and their colors are bright and clear in a well-balanced and healthy individual.

Every chakra regulates the body's various aspects. The root chakra at the base of your spine is associated with the red color and regulates your sense of security. The root chakra forms the foundation of your relationship with the universe. It's also the same as the instinct for life. A blocked root chakra can cause financial uncertainty, anxiety, lack of trust, and even basic food and shelter problems.

The 2nd chakra, known as the Sacral chakra, is found in the abdomen and is connected to the orange color. It regulates relationships, sexuality, imagination, ingenuity, and fertility-related matters. You can find that clearing this chakra will work miracles if you have relationship issues.

The 3rd chakra, the chakra of the Solar Plexus, is at the base of the rib cage and is defined by the yellow color. This chakra is often called the chakra of power, as it is linked to self-worth, intelligence, trust, and strength. When blocked, this chakra can cause you to feel frustrated with the lack of power or control and may even make you feel cynical, negative or overly analytical.

The fourth chakra, the chakra of the heart, is the core of the energetic body and regulates the love emotion. Blockages can make one feel insecure, unloved and even bitter or jealous in this chakra. The chakra of the heart is essential because the lower chakras are linked to the upper chakras. The chakra of the heart is defined by the green color and is located in front of the chest.

The color blue is the 5th chakra, the throat chakra, and it lies in the region of the throat. Chakra allows us to express ourselves and provides us with good communication skills. People with blockages in this chakra can experience communication difficulties or even chronic colds.

The 6th chakra, the third eye or brow chakra is just above the eyebrows in the middle of the forehead. This chakra is defined by the indigo color and reflects the intuitive vision and our relation to the realm of the spirit. This chakra allows us to imagine our intuition and improve it. Blockages can cause confusion, poor concentration, and even headaches in this chakra.

At the top of the head is the 7th chakra, the crown chakra, depicted by the color violet and white. The chakra of the crown leads us to higher guidance and gives us spiritual awareness and is our link to a higher power.

Clearing the chakras will relieve blockages and many techniques can be used; meditation is just one of those methods. By visualizing the color of each chakra spinning clockwise in front of your head, you will clear the chakras and take time to visualize emotional problems clearing up as the colors spin.

Meditation is an incredible way to heal your mind and body, and taking time to work through each chakra will help you solve problems you've been battling for a lifetime.

Meditations are incredibly powerful and can support you in every way to transform your life. Meditation is much more than it meets the eye, and something like meditation has many psychological benefits. Meditation provides you with an escape from reality, and it can also help you live longer, improve the neuroplasticity of your brain, and help you think better. Meditation also helps you release endorphins that are healthy chemicals in your body that make meditation almost as powerful, if not more effective, than common drugs like Prozac!

The Full Chakras of Healing

A chakra is a source of energy in the body, according to Hindu ism. It is at this stage that the strength of the body is highly potent and can be harnessed using appropriate methods.

The term ' chakra' is a wheel-meaning Sanskrit language. Such chakras are often said to be spinning energy plates, found in the subtle body and not the physical body. A stream known as the' Nadi' links the sources or chakras. The fundamental force of life, known as' Prana' in Sanskrit, is believed to be flowing through these Nadis.

The presence of 7 known chakras in the human body is verified by an analysis of ancient scriptures. Apart from the seven essential chakras, there are another 11 chakras, taking the number to 18. These 18 chakras are said to have the ability to heal any illness that the human body faces if properly harnessed.

Let's look at some basic facts about these chakras: • There are seven major chakras and eleven minor chakras.

• All of these chakras are horizontally aligned along the central path.

• They are the powerhouses with the channel (Nadi) and wind (Ardhanarishwara - Vayu Deity (Sanskrit: God - half female, half male. Shiva/Shakti).

• All of them are round in shape and have spokes or petals.

• All of them refer to or are aligned with another god and control a different function of the body.

• The chakras are also referred to as magnetic points in the Western study school and are used to perform the same functions like those listed in the Eastern study school.

• Chakras are not an irrational belief term. Extensive research has been carried out and ample evidence is available to support the existence of such' magnetic points' throughout the human body.

Yoga practitioners, such as the renowned Yoga Guru, B.K.S Iyengar, have often been called upon to address the medical importance of these chakras. The importance of these chakras has been studied in-depth with the help of people like Guru Iyengar.

Let's move on to this section 's main subject, which is the 18 Chakras of Life and their Healing Power.

A list of the 18 chakras is given below according to their location in the human body, their respective roles and how they promote healing.

1. Sahasrara (Thousand-petaled Sanskrit) Place-Head crown or above the head crown.

Color-White God-Dhruva The Sahasrara Chakra is often referred to as the chakra of basic life. It is said to be the highest energy source that begins flowing from the top of the head. This functions like the pituitary gland. The hypophyseal gland secretes hormones to interact with all other endocrine systems and regulates the central nervous system as well. Likewise, the Sahasrara chakra's energy passes through the central nervous system from the top of the head and enters the next chakra through the brain, via a Nadi.

This helps bring harmony to life.

2. Ajna (Command Sanskrit) Place-between the brows of the head. Color-Blue Deity-Ardhanarishwara (Sanskrit: God-half male, half female. Shiva / Shakti) Ajna Chakra, positioned like the third eye, between the eyebrows. This is traditionally part of Hindu mythology, where, when in extreme rage, Lord Shiva, the destroyer of evil, was ordered to open his third eye. When the Lord opened his third eye, it burned to ashes all that fell on his road.

Fun fact, the entire third-eye that burns things to ashes is often said to be the reason Lord Shiva is depicted as an ascetic. Over long periods, he meditated to control his frustration. So he was usually a calm person. But when he got upset, well, dust to dust, ashes to ashes!

Nevertheless, the Ajna chakra deals with a higher intuitive level offering clarity. It's the very focus of attention. In reality, when practicing pranayama (breathing control) in yoga, people are always told to concentrate on the Ajna chakra and keep it as their concentration core. It helps increase the period of attention and gives an excellent ability to concentrate.

3. Vishuddha (Sanskrit for' particularly pure') Location — Throat (parallel to Thyroid) Color — Pale blue or Turkish Deity— Dyaus The Vishuddha chakra is associated with interaction and creation. It is about speech, whether it is spoken, written or not. The location near the thyroid gland, responsible for growth and maturation, further explains the importance of this environment.

This chakra also helps to control speech and modulate sound. This is why the chanting of the sacred' Om' is done in a way that reverberates in the throat while doing Yoga. This activates the chakra and increases energy levels.

4. Anahata (Sanskrit for' unstruck') Location — middle of chest color — green or pink Deity— Ishana Rudra Shiva The Anahata chakra is connected to the thymus, an item in the chest that is part of both the immune and endocrine system and the site of T-cells maturation.

T-cells are the cells that help the infection fight against the body. So Anahata or Unstruck was aptly called. Because of its similarity to the body, it is also called the heart chakra. This deals with energy flow associated with complex compassion, empathy, emotions, etc. Sanskrit for Jewel City

5.(Manipura) Location-Navel or close pancreas Color-Yellow Deity-Agni Manipura is one of the important chakras as it deals with pancreatic and adrenaline functions. It is correlated with the basic digestive process, which is probably the most essential, as digestion transforms food matter into energy.

The chakra deals with the power of this kind. It also deals with the spirit of speech at an emotional level. Perhaps why they're saying' No balls, no glory!

6. Svadhisthana (Sanskrit for one's base) Place-Sacrum Color-White Deity-Bramha This chakra is active mainly

in testes or ovaries. This controls the flow of energy through the sexual organs, enabling the organs to be powerful in reproduction.

The Deity associated with this Chakra, if you may have heard, is Bramha.

Lord Bramha was the Creator or progenitor of creation, according to Hinduism. Therefore, it seems almost fitting to link this organ with none other than the proposed life-giver!

Reproduction, friendships and also addictions are the key issues that the Svadhisthana chakra deals with. It is meant to be the human' urges ' driven and regulated by this chakra.

7. Muladhara (Sanskrit for Root Support) Place— Spine Color Base — Red Deity— Ganesh It is linked to the fundamental human capacity, protection, and survival. Some injuries to the spinal cord, as we all know, can cause permanent damage or even death to the central nervous system.

Therefore, naming this chakra the Muladhara or Root Aid is fitting.

The value of this chakra is that it regulates stability—emotional, physical, psychological, and all other stability forms.

This is where you get the expression "Need a backbone!" The last point of the Nadi is often named, where the energy source stops and the process is repeated.

Let's look at the 11 minor chakras now that we've explored the 7 major chakras. Please note that these are the main chakras. These are aided by the remaining 11 chakras.

8. Hridhaya The Hridhaya chakra is essentially the chakra from which the pulse is said to resonate, situated 2 finger spaces to the left of the Anahata Chakra and then 2 fingers down.

This assists the chakra of the Anahata and helps to regulate the heart's rhythm by the proper flow of energy.

9. Hidden Chakras (Goleta, Lalata, Lalana) The nineth, tenth and eleventh chakras, namely the Goleta, Lalata and Lalana Chakras, are in harmony with the Vishuddha chakra at the back of the throat. We monitor the palette as well as the stream of energy from the chakra through the throat by Nadi.

12. Atala-at the bottom of the hip, controls fear and desire

13. Located in the hip, Vitala controls anger and resentment

14. Located in the thighs, Sutala regulates envy

15. Found in calves, Talatala controls sustained willfulness

16. Rasatala-located in the feet, core of egoism and

17 animal instinct. Mahakala-located in the feet, without awareness, considered the domain

18. Patala-located in the sole, the domain of evil, torture, murder, etc. The chakras from the 12th to the 18th are part of the chakra portion of Muladhara. They dropped below the chakra of Muladhara and are therefore considered to be the least or lesser chakras.

Such 18 chakras together form Healing's 18 chakras. The strength of these 18 chakras can be harnessed by yoga, Pranayam, kundalini, etc. Once these chakras are in harmony, they have the power to heal from within, any pain that one may feels. We are the source of spiritual energy in the human body.

CHAPTER THREE:
Psychic Development - Using Chakras to Aid Psychic Awareness

Anyone is said to be a little psychic, they simply don't know. We all have a specific way of seeing the truth of things, and we each have a special way of interpreting the world around us because we are all different. Our perception approaches are largely based on intuitive assessments. Psychic insight is a skill-based on perception. One must learn how to build on their intuitive abilities to improve one's psychic ability. Operating with your chakras is one of those processes. The chakras are your entire body's energy centers. Such centers are universal energy conduits. That fundamental force provides the link between the higher mind and your consciousness.

Psychic insight is a consequence of balanced centers of energy and connectivity. Most psychic readers may understand the effect of some greater power in their psychic perception which helps them. We often become messengers of divine wisdom for their bodies and minds. While they may not be conscious of it, most definitely their chakras promote their experience. Chakra in Sanskrit means "the wheel." Each chakra, consisting of pure energy, spins into its vibration cycle. Like a wheel, to obtain and release energy, the chakras turn at different speeds. As they allow spiritual power to pass through them, they are portals of psychic energy. Throughout the body, there are seven big chakras. Each chakra is aligned against the spine with a position. It is almost important to note that a corresponding endocrine gland is present in each chakra. The body plays a major role in the development of psychology. It's important to work in harmony with your energy centers and endocrine system. Balancing your body by opening your chakras will make spiritual information flow possible. I listed the seven major chakras in your body below. It is important to recognize that chakras provide you with psychic knowledge to begin deepening your abilities as a psychic reader.

1st Chakra: Our physical body is regulated by the root chakra. Located at the base of the spine, the root chakra is the slowest vibrating chakra connected to our survival instincts. The root chakra is psychologically linked to our self-image and safety feelings. Since the gonads are the correlating glandular attachment, our sex drive and primary impulses are welcomed by the root chakra. In the pelvic area, this chakra energy is mainly focused. We can give and receive sexual pleasure when this chakra is balanced. This chakra also has to do with fertility.

2nd Chakra: Holy Chakra Attached to the root chakra is the holy chakra. It is situated below the naval a few fingers. Sexuality and reproduction are linked to the sacral chakra. Your physical well-being may be at risk when this chakra is out of control. The sacral chakra reflects the life force when it is accessible and protected. We're looking for a physical union with someone from this power. It is linked to the adrenal and lymphatic system. The adrenaline in your body is activated when agitated, maintaining the body in an alert state. It taxes the body and if its power destroys the holy chakra. Working with this chakra when stressed is necessary. It can help calm the nervous system by controlling this chakra. Emotionally, this chakra has to do with our well-being emotions and feelings. This chakra encourages clarification in terms of chakras that support the psychic reader. Clairsentience is a form of touch-related psychic ability. This allows the ability of a psychic reader to hold an object or touch someone and to feel the energy that surrounds that person, place or thing.

3rd Chakra: Solar Plexus The chakra of the solar plexus applies to our strength and digestion rates. It's situated between the bridge and the naval. Emotionally, our perceptions of personal power in the world are discussed by the solar plexus. It also helps in a healthy ego's growth. The pancreas and adrenal glands are associated with it. If this chakra is out of control, there is a risk that the proper functioning of one's stomach, liver and/or pancreas. This is also a spiritual energy-promoting chakra. This refers to a "second sight" in this situation, the same power with which mediums operate. Opening this chakra helps a psychic reader to increase their knowledge of the paranormal. This chakra promotes prophetic visions and spiritual insight. We get "happy" feelings from this chakra.

4th Chakra: The Heart Chakra is found between your shoulder blades in the middle of your heart. The chakra of the heart is linked to the Universal Mind. This contributes psychologically to affection and sincerity. Physically, the heart and lungs are regulated by the heart chakra. This controls the thymus as well. There is a chance of immune defects and heart problems when out of control. Compassion and kindness to others may also be missing. This is the connectivity chakra. This influences, among others, how you feel. It also impacts your self-esteem and self-love feelings.

5th Chakra: Throat The chakra of the throat is about interaction, imagination and personal growth. Located at the top of the throat, thyroid, head, ears, nose, and mouth are dominated by the throat chakra. Clairaudience is the 5th chakra's strength. Clairaudience allows one to receive messages from another frequency or domain in the form of thoughts. This is regarded as a form of channeling. This chakra psychologically corresponds with the manifestation of one's emotions. When available, it helps to communicate verbally and mentally with others. This is also the logic and reason chakra. You may have sore throats, imaginative barriers, and miscommunications when you are open.

6th Chakra: Third Eye Located in the center of your forehead between your eyebrows, the third eye chakra refers to your pituitary gland, your ears, and your sinuses. This chakra also has to do with one's ability to view and process information. The Third Eye Chakra helps abstract thought to be done. It also helps us to understand the spirit world. It is the consciousness and perception of chakra. The third eye chakra psychologically reflects tolerance and acceptance. The third eye chakra, at the same time, is a force that pushes us forward. This chakra, once open, helps us to communicate our wishes and assume responsibility for our choices. The Third Eye Chakra encompasses how we interpret things in terms of psychic abilities, including the emotions and feelings of others. It also helps us to increase our understanding of the extrasensory. The third eye chakra allows them to see the bigger picture of things for the psychic reader. It's a talent called clear-sightedness. This is the capacity to see objects in the lens of the brain.

7th Chakra: Crown The crown chakra is on the top of the head. This chakra is connected with one's universe relation. It is the chakra of consciousness and the crown chakra will not work in full capacity until the other six chakras are balanced. This is the highest vibrating chakra that meets the strength and reality of God. This helps one to receive messages from the divine spirit when open. The crown chakra gives the understanding of the unknown to a spiritual writer. If the crown chakra is blocked, psychological problems like anxiety or depression can be felt. It has to do with the thalamus. Recognizing that each individual has a unique way to work with their chakras is significant.

No "one" way or "wrong" way is possible. It's a personal experience and process. If you have never tried to balance your chakras, you may want to experiment with some guided meditations that will take you through your energy center opening process. I considered this quite helpful. Do not be surprised if you work with your chakras and you find yourself opening up to new spiritual skills. Trust the ride and enjoy it.

How Chakras Function in the Physical Body

The concept of chakras is derived from an ancient yoga scheme. The word chakra comes from Sanskrit and means "disk" or "plate," but it typically implies a circle of power. The old Indian theologians considered a chakra hub of the bodies as fluttering, axle-like vortices of energy. This section will give you a synopsis of the chakras in the human body and their work. When you know how each chakra influences your physical function, you can better determine which chakra can be blocked or congested, then work to improve the chakra.

There are seven major chakras from the base of the spine to the top of the head, aligned horizontally up and down the spine, within the physical body. Around the spine, endocrine system, and numerous glands, they are connected to the nervous system. The chakras are also associated with various functions of the body, such as breathing and digestion.

Essentially, the seven main chakras reflect the four elements— earth, water, flame, and air — as well as sound, light, and thought. Growing chakra has one of the rainbow's seven colors— red, orange, yellow, green, blue, indigo, and violet. The numerous organs and glands in the body are also connected with these centers. A description of the numerous chakras— their color, place, and physical function in our body follows.

First Chakra–Red: The Red Root Center is the first chakra. It is at the base of the spine and is connected to our physical body and behavior. Reproductive organ, uterus, prostate, adrenal glands, spinal column, tailbone, teeth, ribs, arms, and feet are regulated by the Root Chakra.

Second Chakra— Orange: Spleen Chakra is the second chakra and orange. Lung Chakra found in the pubic area and is responsible for spleen, ovaries, testes, uterus, kidneys, and urinary organs.

Third Chakra— Yellow: The Solar Plexus or 3rd Chakra is yellow and linked to our self of mind and thought. There're two chakras of the Solar Plexus the other in the back and one in front, externally regulating the heart, liver, gallbladder, pancreas, sympathetic nervous system, intestines, digestive system and blood sugar.

Fourth Chakra— Green: the fourth Heart Chakra is in color green. There are two chakras again, one in the middle of the chest in front of the physical heart and the other in the back. This means both the front and back chakras as they refer to the Heart Chakra. The Heart Chakra physically regulates the heart, gland of thymus, lungs, bronchia, lymph system, secondary circulatory system, immune system, legs, and feet.

Fifth Chakra— Blue: The fifth chakra is the blue chakra of the Throat Chakra. The thyroid, parathyroid, hypothalamus, stomach, chest, jaw, and mouth are physically regulated by this chakra.

Sixth— Indigo: The Brow is the sixth chakra located in the area between the eyebrows and its color is indigo. The third eye is also named because it is related to our common self-seeing. The pituitary gland, cerebellum (lower brain), head, nose, ears, and nervous system are physically regulated by this chakra.

Seventh Chakra— Violet: The Crown is the seventh chakra and is colored violet. This chakra is at the head's crown. The pineal gland, cerebral cortex (upper brain), central nervous system, and skin are physically regulated by the Crown Chakra.

As you can see, the physical operation of each chakra is different. Therefore, each chakra also affects your personality. Your physical, emotional and spiritual bodies will benefit if the chakras are consistent and balanced. Chakra clearing can be a great tool for better health and well-being.

Connecting Your Chakras Using Reiki

For Reiki 1, binding the Chakras focuses on healing one chakra at a time. When you develop more energy tolerance, you will begin a more complex pattern of healing. Determine the chakras need to be energized by scanning or using a pendulum. Place one hand on the soft chakra and place for 1 to 3 minutes the other hand on the chakra above it. It transfers the power of a stronger chakra to elevate the weaker's strength. Keep your hand on the weak chakra while pushing one more chakra up the other hand until it stabilizes the core. Do this above for every chakra, all the way to the crown.

Link the poor chakra to all the underlying chakras. Hold one hand on the weak chakra and put the other hand on each of the underlying chakras until all the chakras are linked to the weak one. Review this example to link the heart chakra to the upper chakras to summarize the procedure.

Left hand on heart, right hand over throat Left hand over heart, right hand over brow Left hand over heart, right hand over crown Now attach the chakra of heart to the lower chakras.

hand from left on solar, hand from right heart plexus Hand over heart, left hand over sacral chakra Right hand above heart, left hand over root chakra It extends the human heart related to other six chakras, extracting energy from them. Consider the following consequences when linking chakras. For example, when connecting the heart chakra of your patient to other chakras, questions like these can direct your therapeutic communication: what do you want to communicate about your emotions (chakra 4) (chakra 5)?

How about your creative expression (chakra 5) do you think (chakra 4)?

* ** How about your behavior (chakra 3) do you think (chakra 4)?

What can you do to fix your thoughts (chakra 4) (chakra 3)?

* ** Chakra link can be a strong way to complete your character. You will have a better idea of your strengths and weaknesses after studying the characteristics of each of the chakras. For example, when you consider your solar plexus overloaded as demonstrated by very high self-confidence and a highly driven personality, this indicates excess energy in your third chakra.

When you find at the same time that your reproductive system includes cysts or tumors, it indicates a low or closed second chakra. Determine -chakras are most in need of healing and interaction by examining your traits and physical symptoms.

Chakra Spread For extreme emotional or physical distress this technique is used. This takes a person further than most other strategies to a healing level. Special needs and special healing times should be reserved. Tell your client to sit while you stand in front of them in a chair. Start by being well-rooted, mentally stable, and physically well connected to the planet. Place your hands for one or two minutes on your patient's feet to make sure they're well-grounded. Then hold the hands of your client is yours to open their palm chakras for one or two minutes. Put both hands on their crown chakra and walk behind your client. Open your crown chakra by raising your hands gently and slowly as far as you can reach, like an eagle's wings. Three times execute this movement. If you need to open other chakras, distribute them in the same way.

The most successful way to approach this material is to revisit it from time to time, but during your healings be careful not to over-intellectualize it. Place each chakra with your hands and let the energy flow. It indicates that if thoughts or images come to mind, your instinct acts to tell you how to proceed. If your mind is still quiet, it's perfect! As my Reiki Master Danielle also tells her students, during each healing release all expectations. Just let the flow of energy. If required, this technical information is always available for further reference on each of the chakras.

CHAPTER FOUR:
The Dynamic System of Chakras

We will concentrate on the complex definition of chakras in this post. To clarify, virtually all references to opening, calming, healing, energizing, clearing or meditating on the chakras apply to the complex concept rather than the yogic/tantric concept. Such two principles as elements of a single system are quite different and incompatible. Most of the chakras ' writings and explanations combine elements from each of these two distinct chakras principles indiscriminately. Most of the data is just a continuation of the same misunderstandings and misunderstandings.

The argument I want to make here is that chakras' experience and understanding come from a relativity system. So if we look at two respected and contemporary exponents of chakra theories such as Barbara Ann Brennan and, for example, Carolyn Myss, we find similarities as well as significant differences. This doesn't mean that one is right and the other is wrong, it's just an example of the chakras ' human experience's relativity. Research and systematology for both of these people have value and legitimacy. They both viewed the chakras ' complex energy system from their individual perception's unique perspective.

Start by mentioning the complex system's seven key chakras as widely agreed. Spread from top to bottom around the body's main nerve plexuses.

Chakra center seven — Crown Chakra center six — 3rd eye— forehead Chakra center five— throat Chakra center four — heart center three — Chakra center two solar plexus— navel center one — perineum But what are the chakras doing? And how is that? Barbara Ann Brennan's view is that "the chakras act as energy intake organs from the universal energy field...... the energy taken in and metabolized through each chakra is sent to the parts of the body located in the nearest region of the median nerve plexus." While Caroline Myss says "every thought and experience you have ever had in your life is transmitted through these chakra databases. We can also see them as a vibrational scale, from the lowest vibrational frequencies in the base chakra to the highest vibrational frequencies in and beyond the Crown chakra. Nevertheless, it is not my knowledge that the spiritual cycle follows an ascending chakra clearing from base to crown. In many interactions between the various centers, the karmic forces kept in the unconscious are intertwined and interwoven.

For example, a clearing process may start in the second chakra weaving through the heart, the throat, before going down at the solar plexus to the third chakra. This is because, from multiple dimensions of practice, karmic energies can be shaped and retain various levels of vibrational frequency. Also, from my many years of experience doing healing work, the heart chakra is almost always affected, and a catalyst in the healing process.

Barbara Ann Brennan is exceptional in attributing various qualities to the two to six chakras ' front and rear power vortices. Feeling centers are in her complex chakra template a front funnel of two to five chakras. The two to five middle rear funnel is going to point. So psychological centers are both the front and back of the six chakras along with the crown chakra.

The seven main dynamic chakras The first or foundation chakra, found between sex and anus, is associated with the first energy field or aura surface. These contribute to automated and autonomous functioning as well as sensory and emotional perception functioning. This relates directly to the desire to live, to be' here' in the body, on earth, and to physical survival problems.

The second chakra, hara or sacral is found below the belly-button region and is connected to the aura's second layer. The thoughts, desires, sensuality, and sexuality are associated with them. This is the core of personal power, a picture of oneself, and wealth. It is then easy to see how sexuality-power-self-image and money become so confusingly entangled.

The fourth, solar plexus chakra, found in the opening of the lower ribs predictably around the area of the solar plexus, is connected to the third layer of the aura. Both are associated with will, the lower mind for rational and linear thought. This carries the self-image and self-esteem psychological dimension. This chakra is deeply linked to the nervous system, as this is the primary place in the body to retain terror.

The heart chakra located at or above the breastbone level in the middle of the chest is connected to the fourth layer of the aura. We are associated with all facets of love and compassion and higher will emergence. This chakra stands at the core of our being, it houses our humanity's essence and the meeting of spirit and body.

The throat chakra is located above the throat hollow, relates to the fifth layer of the aura, and is associated with the transmission of truth, interaction, and Divine will. It is here that we are witnessing private will surrender.

The sixth brow chakra, located just above the eye level in the middle of the forehead, refers to the aura's sixth surface. Color, subconscious mind, and psychic intuition are correlated with them. Here's a conceptualizing power, it's the seat of the higher mind and imagination.

At the top of the head, the crown chakra is connected to the seventh layer of the aura, they are aligned with spiritual and direct awareness relation. It is the location of the personality's religious integration.

I hope it is clear at this point that the comparisons with the various chakras above are not conclusive at all. You'll note I didn't assign colors, crystals, etc. Alternatively, I encourage you to learn for yourself and discover it. You can find your perception changes over time. Just as every person on the planet is special, so is it in every chakra. So I encourage you again to explore with an open mind, to use your sense and feeling, where a particular crystal could resonate in you, for example, should you be so inclined. Remember that life itself is a dynamic process, constantly moving, and with it, our dynamic chakras are moving constantly.

Wellness of Personal Power of Chakras

Chakra will improve your health and strength.

Before you bring balance to universe, you have to gain stability. You have to open all your Chakras to master your destiny and inner energy, and only then will you know your destiny.

Chakras are like the sea flowing through the swirling pools of the tide, much like the water flowing through the body. Life is messy at times. At certain points you will see the water rising and swirling, objects often emerging to the ocean causing an interference, barrier or blockage in the stream of these energies. It is necessary to open up this problem of gathering mass, stationary energy and increasing pressure at certain points because of the block to allow the energy to flow freely. Chakras are like pools in our bodies that accumulate and spiral heat. If nothing else were around then the water would flow freely with transparency and purity through these spirals of ocean energy.

Opening all the Chakras is necessary, essential so that they can flow in a healthy and harmonious state. There are seven chakras, each one with meaning.

The Earth / Root First Chakra-located at the base of the spine. This Chakra is about survival and fear-blocked. - What are you most afraid of -let your fears be clear to you-surrender these fears-let your fears spill into the ocean Root Chakra Exercises— exercise your root chakra by walking, jumping, and moving the feet to the ground, marching, squatting, and Plyometric.

Feeding vegetables from the Root Chakra Root: carrots, onions, parsnips, radishes, beets, garlic, etc.

Protein: Soy products, pork, eggs, rice, fish, tofu, peas, peanut butter Spices: spicy paprika, horseradish, cayenne, chives, jalapeño, tabasco, pepper, habanera The second chakra This chakra deals with enjoyment and is prevented by remorse. at all the shame that consumes your soul-what are you guilty of accepting the reality of these things, but don't let them cloud or corrupt your power. You must first forgive yourself if you are to be a good influence on the world.

Sacred Chakra Stretches-Exercise the sacred chakra with glute stretches, pelvic thrusts, leg lifts and circular motions of the pelvis.

Nice fruits: melons, bananas, mangos, strawberries, fruits of love, oranges, coconut, etc.

Honey, molasses, nuts from maple syrup: almonds, walnuts, peanuts, nuts from macadamia, etc.

Spices: cinnamon, chocolate, carob, sweet paprika, sesame seeds, caraway seeds The Third Chakra Fire — found in the stomach This Chakra deals with will power and is thwarted by guilt— what are you most ashamed of — what are your biggest disappointments in yourself. Abdomen Chakra Exercises-Exercise the chakra of the abdomen by doing abdominals, diaphragm exercises, spinning, jumping jacks, flipping, hula-hooping, and dancing of the belly.

Granola and grains of the Stomach Chakra: pasta, bread, cereals, beans, flax seeds, seeds of sunflower, etc.

Dairy: milk, cheeses, chocolate, gelato Spices: ginger, peppermint, spearmint, chamomile, turmeric, cumin, fennel The Fourth Chakra-This Chakra deals with love and is blocked by sorrow -Lay out all your sadness before you -Identify any great loss your heart feels Love is a form of energy. All around us it swirls. The air in and out of which Nomads breathed is still left for you and has not left the world. It swirls inside you. It is within your heart and in the form of more love and new love it is reborn.

Heart Chakra Exercises-Pushups, neck exercises, swimming, jumping jacks, yoga, and hugging yourself to strengthen your heart chakra.

Feeding vegetables from the Heart Chakra Leafy: lettuce, kale, lard greens, etc.

Air vegetables: broccoli, sprouts from Brussels, cauliflower, cabbage, celery, onions, etc.

Liquids: green teas, ginseng tea Spices: basil, ginger, thyme, cilantro, parsley Sweets: dark chocolate The fifth chakra This chakra is in the throat This chakra deals with honesty and is distorted by lies-blocked by the lies we tell ourselves You cannot lie about your own identity you should believe that you are the person you know yourself to be.

Throat Chakra Exercises-Gargle your throat chakra with saltwater, humming, singing, or even yelling.

Feeding the throat Chakra Liquids in general: milk, fruit juices, herbal teas Sweet and tangy fruits: lemons, limes, grapefruits, kiwi Tree rising fruits: apples, oranges, plums, peaches, apricots, pineapples Spices: salt, lemongrass The Sixth Chakra This is the Light Chakra located in the center of the forehead This Chakra deals with wisdom and is obscured by delusion-the main illusion of the Chakra. In reality, things that you think are separate and different are the same. We're all one person, but we're living as if separated. All of us are related. It's all linked. An example; an illusion is even the separation of the elements. The elements are all one. The pieces of the same whole are the elements.

Light Chakra Exercises-With imagining, creativity, conscious thought, remote viewing, and lucid dreaming, exercise the light chakra.

Feeding the light-dark bluish fruits of the Chakra: blueberries, red grapes, blackberries, raspberries, strawberries, etc.

Liquids: red wines and grape juice Spices: lavender, poppy seed The Seventh Chakra This is the Chakra of Thinking and is found on the head's crown. This Chakra deals with pure cosmic energy and the earthly connection prevents it. Think about what's connecting you to this planet. Now, let go of all the attachments during meditation. Let them float forgotten into the sea. Learn to let go or you won't let the pure divine energy float out of the universe and can't.

Crown Chakra Exercises-Train the crown chakra by reading, exploring, praying and/or meditating.

Feeding The Crown Chakra Incense and Smudging Herbs: Tea, Copal, Myrrh, Incense, and Juniper You must open all the Chakras to master yourself. Give up yourself. You have to open all your chakras and only then will you understand your destiny, have complete mastery, control and knowledge of all your actions.

How to use Chakra Meditation When You Feel Blocked

Meditation with chakras is a good way to enhance your well-being and well-being. You shift your power by doing chakra meditation. Not only do you feel better when you shift your power, but it can also help you move forward more easily on your journey.

That's why meditation on chakras can be good if you feel somehow blocked. Keeping clean and flowing your energy lets you connect to a higher vibration level. Your Self and the World (God, Higher Source, etc.) interact more easily as the world does not have to go through all the energy muck produced in your energy system.

A Short Description of Chakras and Chakra Meditation The Sanskrit word ' chakra' means' bar' or' disk.' These are spherical, funnel-shaped centers of energy that are believed to be in the etheric body of matter also called the subtle body.

The etheric body is the non-physical body that our material bodies are superimposed over. It is an exact copy of our physical body but in a higher form of energy. It can be measured as the electromagnetic fields in and around everything.

Chakras transfer energy to the physical body. We even transmit the vibration of our feelings, emotions, and physical health into the energy field around us. Looking at the chakras and aura of a person will give you a glimpse of what they might feel or how well their emotions and physical body function.

I found the difference chakra meditation can bring in my students ' energy system. When I teach people to do chakra meditation, there is a tangible difference that I can sense from before and after chakra meditation in their energy and sometimes in the energy of the room. I can see the difference in their chakras before and after mentally.

Most generally, chakras are symbolized as cones of power whirling or petalled flowers. Chakras have openings on both the front and back of the etheric organ, except the crown (pointing up) and root (pointing down) chakras with one opening.

First Chakras Used in Traditional Chakra Meditations Seven main chakras are known to be associated with the spine. These are the ones that most mp3s concentrate on chakra meditation. The first chakra, the Root Chakra, binds us to the earth and is about our roots and friends. This is also where, if we are steady and on our feet, we feel safe and secure.

Common name: Root Chakra, Base Chakra Sanskrit name: Muladhara (meaning Support) Location: Spine base, Perineum The Root Chakra is a red cone of energy pointing down to earth. The red is visualized as bright and vibrant as possible in a chakra meditation and reaches down between the legs from the perineum.

The second chakra, the sacral chakra, is associated with the influence of feminine energy (both male and female) and imagination.

Common name: Sacral Chakra, Splenic Chakra (this chakra is situated above the spleen in some Eastern systems) Sanskrit name: Svadhisthana (meaning sweetness) Location: lower abdomen, about two inches below the navel The sacral chakra is colored orange. There are two cones of fuel-one coming out in the body's front and one in the body's back. You can think of a ripe orange in a chakra meditation to help you imagine the richness of the orange color.

The third chakra, the chakra of the solar plexus, is the center of determination, the center of personal power, self-esteem, self-worth. This is the same field where the intuitive insight of the mind and intuition of the brain is received.

Common name: Solar Plexus Chakra Sanskrit name: Manipura (meaning Lustrous Pearl, or Navel Jewel) Location: Solar plexus, upper abdomen, below the breastbone, about two inches above the navel The solar plexus chakra is bright yellow. It has two power cones, one at the back and one at the front. Consider about the sun and how bright yellow it is in a chakra trance. This is how vividly you want your solar plexus chakra to be visualized.

The fourth chakra, the chakra of the soul, is where we keep affection-for others and ourselves. Compassion and forgiveness are created here. Happiness brings us into contact with others and the world.

Common name: Heart Chakra Sanskrit Name: Anahata (meaning Unbeaten or Unstuck) Location: Chest core The heart chakra is painted as emerald green or purple. It has two power cones, one at the back and one at the front. Whether pink or smaragd green is perfect in chakra meditation. None of them are stronger than the other. It's what for you resonate.

The fifth chakra, the throat chakra, is about the ability to express oneself, to be imaginative and to connect. This chakra is correlated with psychic vision and clairaudience.

Common name: Throat Chakra Sanskrit name: Visshudha (meaning purification) Location: throat middle The throat chakra is blue sky. It has two power cones, one at the back and one at the front. You want to make the blue a rich sky blue or the blue you see in the Caribbean waters in chakra meditation. Please do not have baby blues or pastels.

Third Eye Chakra Chakra six is our source of inner vision, creativity, and intuition, the third eye chakra. It is where we can control clear-sightedness or see mentally.

Common name: Third Eye or Brow Chakra Sanskrit name: Ajna (meaning Perceive or Command) Location: middle of the forehead (not the middle of eyebrows) The color of your 3rd eye chakra is indigo. It has two power cones, one at the back and one at the front. Think of the midnight-blue sky in a chakra meditation to aid you with indigo light.

The seven Crown Chakra Chakra binds us to our higher self, higher consciousness, and the universe's divine knowledge.

Common name: Crown Chakra Sanskrit Name: Sahasrara (meaning Thousandfold or Thousand-Petalled lotus) Location: Top of the neck, slightly forward The crown chakra is painted in violet, white or gold. There is one power cone that extends downwards.

Why are Chakras Blocked Up?

You're a good being. There's also strength in your thoughts and emotions. Chakras get clogged with dark-looking, sluggish, heavy energy when we have thoughts and emotions full of self-criticism, prolonged anger, prolonged shame— all the negative types of energies we normally try to avoid falling into.

The way your chakras work can also be influenced by your physical body. Your feelings, emotions, and physical health are all commonly believed to be interconnected.

I've seen sick people with a turbid, soft, tiny and cloudy energy system. I also saw chakras in different health conditions— from being tiny and usually bright to oddly shaped, dull in color, enormous and bright, light and cheerful, dark and heavy.

These are all manifestations of the state of mind, feelings, and physical health of the person. Negative emotions, unhealthy foods, stress, being surrounded by negative people-all these factors will begin to affect the value of your energy vibration.

Those tend to be a lower frequency, slower energy waves that can be absorbed and carried into your energy system. When this happens, it begins to mess with how energy can be stored by your chakras. That's when chakras get confused and may continue to get blocked.

Why Chakra Meditation Works Chakra Meditation uses your mind's power and visualization ability to change your focus. The power can be influenced by your brain.

Chakra meditation helps you stay focused on your mind and guides you through each chakra. You are directed in the meditation to perceive each chakra.

Sometimes I have students who are having trouble seeing or are working to open up their clear-sighted skills. That's all right if you can't see the chakras mentally.

You don't have to be active for you to have chakra meditation. I ask my students in these situations to think, visualize what their chakras look like, or just know what that particular chakra is like.

You think that's perfect though. In clearing your chakras, it is the purpose and concentration that is relevant.

It can be done daily or whenever you think you need to do the chakra meditation that I offer people. You don't even need to use the mp3 anymore once you get into the routine, even though some people like being driven through it.

When you find that there is one particular chakra that is more difficult to visualize or takes longer to clear, it means that the energy field has a certain resistance. Sometimes it is a conviction that we cling to stubbornly about ourselves or the universe. Some times it's because we generally ignore our relaxation needs.

You may want to pick up some colorful paint chips if you have difficulty visualizing the hue, one for each chakra color and have it with you for chakra meditation. As you need, you can use them as a guide.

CHAPTER FIVE:
Cosmic Focuses Of Energy with Chakra Malas

All of us are energy beings and part of this magnificent world. The chakra colors or the body's seven celestial energy centers are aligned with the rainbow colors: orange, indigo, violet, brown, blue, yellow, red. Just as all colors are merged into the purest white of the thousand-petalled loti, so too are the energy centers balanced to achieve our ultimate consciousness. In the field of human life, chakras are key celestial focuses on energy. Located along the body's central path from the base of the spine to the highest point of the head, chakras are essential prana concentrations that are always in motion, matching the energies with the universe's auras.

Violet is the color of the Crown chakra, also known as Sahasrara with the brilliance of the moon as the seat of eternal consciousness. Where the breath of life merges into Shiva's limitless world. This chakra is at the head's highest point. The chakra of the Crown is linked to the crown of the head, the sensory system, and the brain, reflecting pure thought and action, everlasting, Divine life. This chakra links one with the infinite knowledge and the divine origin. Opening this chakra will help leverage a profound spiritual perception where the Shakti and Shiva combine as non-duality. Gemstone mala bead that are the sphatik or transparent quartz that will support the Crown chakra.

Indigo: Brow or Third-Eye chakra shade, otherwise known as Ajna. This chakra is the location of the soul unfolding between the eye temples. We are freed from suffering by knowledge and simple conscious thought. The awakening of the KundalinÄ results in being able to see the actions and those of others without prejudice but with apathy. We are who we are, and we are part of the obvious inclusive. Simple intuition, instinct, trustworthiness can be strengthened by opening this chakra. The Ajna Chakra is connected to the Sapphire Japa mala.

Blue: The color of the Throat chakra, also known as Visuddhi, is connected to purification and equilibrium that can be energized by pranayama or controlled breathing. This chakra is situated in the throat or larynx where sound waves are produced in mantras. Just as mantras are vibrations that are calming and healing, hurtful words harm not only the other but also yourself. Controlling or regulating the throat chakra will result in spiritual purification that will create outlets for great worldly interaction. Opening the chakra of the Throat improves visual vision. Gemstone malas that will add turquoise, blue lapis, sodalite to the Throat chakra.

Green: The color of the chakra of the heart, otherwise called Anahata, where the unconscious is unfolding and a gamut of emotions is present. This chakra is linked to the cardiovascular plexus of the chest, lungs, circulatory systems. The Chakra of the Heart conquers every barrier between the spiritual and the physical universe. Inner Healing leads to understanding and self-knowledge. Opening the chakra of the heart enables a person to have more compassion, understanding, and empathy. Gemstones yoga malas that will help integrate emerald, tourmaline, aventurine, malachite, rose quartz into the heart chakra.

Yellow: Solar Plexus chakra's shadow, also known as Manipura. This chakra is the abode of insight, wisdom, self-confidence, and well-being in the stomach region. Manipuri chakra food and digestion seat is our soul's fire, the sacred energy. Food sensations are carried into our chakras, here we have the power to remove negative thoughts. The chakra of the Solar Plexus reflects imperative action and self-consciousness. Food sensations are carried into our chakras, here we have the power to remove negative thoughts. The chakra of the Solar Plexus reflects imperative action and self-consciousness. This helps a man to find his value when this chakra is open, turning dreams and goals into reality. Gemstone mala beads and bracelets that will add silver, topaz, citrine, green jasper to the Solar Plexus chakra.

Orange: The Sacral Chakra's shadow, also known as Svadhisthana, is the seat of subconsciousness, between sleeping and being awake, and is Karmas ' trigger position. This chakra is between the sacrum and the coccyx. The Sacred Chakra is associated with procreation's sexual organs. Letting go of the past, the ego that holds on to memories and practice of judgment, this is where the kundalini starts to ascend. Opening this chakra will give free will energy and focused action vigor. The Sacred Chakra is associated with procreation's sexual organs. Letting go of the past, the ego that holds on to memories and practice of judgment, this is where the kundalini starts to ascend. Opening this chakra will give free will energy and focused action vigor Gemstone yoga males which help to integrate carnelian, coral, orange jasper, orange jade into the sacral chakra.

Red: The Root Chakra color, otherwise known as Mujadara, the beginning of our spiritual growth. This chakra is located at the base of the spine and helps us to be rooted in a dark, dormant state where the kundalini shakti sleeps. The seat of the unconscious, the root chakra is where we begin to assess our existence and purify the spiritual energy. The seat of the unconscious, the root chakra is where we begin to assess our existence and purify the spiritual energy. Yoga beads and Gemstone mala beads that will attach diamond, hematite, obsidian, Smokey quartz, garnet, and onyx to the Root chakra.

The Affection of on Our Personality

This section will concentrate on what part of your personality the different chakras refer to and two simple strategies for clearing and managing them. The energy centers need to be open and balanced, as this enables the energy to flow freely up and down the spine and throughout the nervous system. The effect is often a sense of peace and well-being as the physical, psychological, emotional and spiritual bodies are directly related to the chakra system. Tension, negative emotions and other unbalanced energies can be released from the chakras that can support the whole individual as there is a link between all the bodies. Because all the chakras are linked when the whole chakra system is affected by one region.

Chakras First Chakra-Red qualities: Motivation, zeal, strength, and grounding are some of the qualities. Red helps give us energy, bravery, inner strength, and self-confidence, and inspires our goals to be accomplished. It gives us the strength and power to fulfill our dreams.

Second Chakra-Orange: It is associated with our psychological and self-feeling, and some of its attributes are pleasure, satisfaction, and socialization.

Third Chakra-Yellow: This is our ego core and some of its attributes are confidence, intellect, and cognitive imagination. This chakra greatly affects the brain.

Fourth Chakra-Green: a hub for energy clearing house is the Solar Plexus Chakra. Upon entering the higher chakras and vice versa, a large portion of energy from the lower chakras is assumed to pass through this front chakra. Through energizing this chakra, the entire body can be enhanced. This chakra is connected to our self of devotion. Harmony, compassion, empathy, emotional balance, unconditional love, understanding, and development are some of its attributes.

Fifth Chakra-Blue: The Chakra of the Throat is connected to our expressive selves. Honesty, politeness, imaginative self-expression and will are some of its attributes. It also helps to prepare and coordinate in-depth.

Sixth Chakra-Indigo: This chakra is also called the master chakra because the other chakras and their related endocrine glands are regulated and managed. It is also called the third eye, as it is related to our fundamental self-seeing. Some of the attributes are wisdom, looking for reality, and intuition.

Seventh Chakra-Violet: This chakra is connected to our spiritual self and awareness. Some of the qualities are creativity, charisma, ability to see life's beauty, and it helps purify thoughts and feelings. It also enhances our desire to be artistic and creative.

There are many methods to clear, align and energize the chakras, but I'm going to give you a few simple ones that anyone can do. First technique: shake hands to remove old strength, then rub your hands together briskly. This stimulates the smaller chakras in your hands and transfers the power. They could feel warm. First, put both hands on the chakra with which you would like to work. Picture universal healing energy coming into your hands as you go about clearing, calming, and energizing the chakra on which you are holding your hands. As this happens, you could feel the heat going into that zone. Continue for a few minutes or until you think it's over. When you are done, shake off the heat. Follow the next chakra's process.

Second Technique: When you lie down, this one could be better. To clear the heat, shake your hands, then rub them together briskly. First, open both palms, palm down, one over the other. Place both hands over the chakra you are working with and begin to rotate about 3 to 4 inches above the chakra in the counterclockwise direction. Make slow counterclockwise circles around one to two minutes over the chakra or until you think it's full.

Then shake your hands for half as long as the counterclockwise motion releases the power and spins clockwise. The movement of the clock soothes and stabilizes the chakra removed. Do the same cycle you are clearing for each chakra. Clear the crown chakra in a clockwise direction for a person to clear and then sooth in a counterclockwise direction. All the remaining chakras are the same as above.

Every day or whenever you feel the need, you can use these techniques. Start with a place where you feel uncomfortable. As mentioned above, each chakra has its personality traits. Look at the specific areas, such as the heart chakra, that cause you discomfort. This cycle can produce harmful or blocked energies that can then pass out of your body. Because we express ourselves through these energy centers, once stress and negative feelings have been released, we can shift into a more balanced state of well-being. Recall that all the chakras are linked, so clearing one will also affect the others. Clearing the chakras will improve the whole system of energy.

Aligning Chakra Points With Chakra Jewelry

The next step in finding your life's ideal chakra jewelry is to know exactly what the chakra points are doing. You can choose each piece of chakra jewelry wisely. While some of each separate chakra's different colors and symbols can appeal to you, it is also important to buy chakra jewelry to help balance any ailing chakra points in your body.

The first level of the chakra is called the Sahasrara. Also named the "Crown Chakra." It is known to be the pure consciousness associated with the chakra. It is considered to be identical to that of the pituitary gland in the operation of the body. To interact with your whole endocrine system, it secretes hormones. Also symbolized with precisely one thousand petals by a beautiful lotus. The chakra of the crown is at the head's "crown." Not only a lotus flower reflects this chakra, but the vivid shade of violet. Of which the force for inner wisdom helps to reflect. Crown chakra jewelry is often considered to help read. Helping others open their minds to the world and their lives are seen.

First, you've got the chakra of Ajna. Often known as the chakra of the third eye. It is thought to be connected to the pineal gland that is known to have the power of imagination. It is understood that the pineal gland is light-sensitive, releasing hormone melatonin to control cycles of sleep and wakefulness. The Ajna is portrayed by a two-petalled lotus. It also displays red, indigo, and blue colors. It is believed that the third eye chakra will aid not only in sleep and wakefulness but will also help you access the many different benefits of intuition, emotion, and clarity. The chakra jewelry that reflects the third eye chakra is created to help in the term of their life "open one's eyes." Allowing them to achieve a balance within themselves and allowing their internal guidance to be accessed and trusted.

Second, you're going to get to know the chakra vishuddha. Also known as "the chakra of the Throats." The thyroid gland is thought to be related. Of which the thyroid hormone is in the mouth. Which is in control of development and maturation. A lotus that has seventeen petals symbolizes it. The throat chakra is shown in pale blue and turquoise colors. Self-expression and interaction are thought to be regulated. That's why the jewelry of the throat chakra will help you communicate with your speech of yourself. It is also often used to help someone conquer public speaking shyness and anxiety.

The fourth chakra is the chakra of the Anahata. Also known as the chakra of the chest. The thymus is associated (located inside the chest). The Thymus is a complex part of the body's endocrine system; it contains t-cells. Whose duty is to ward off illness or disease. Nevertheless, the compounding of daily stress is considered to be adversely affected. A lotus with twelve petals symbolizes the heart chakra. It is often portrayed with bright green and pink colors. Used to help balance one's soul, heart chakra jewelry. Whether it's emotional chaos, passion, or just allowing one's self to conquer heart pain. Helping in love and spirituality is also acknowledged.

It is assumed that the Manipura (Solar Plexus Chakra) or fifth chakra is directly related to the metabolic and digestive system. The solar plexus is said to have a link with the body's energy as well as the ability to help with personal power problems, fear (fear), anxiety, form your own opinions, and switch between simple and complex emotions. A lotus with ten petals, often colored by bright yellow hues, represents the Solar plexus chakra. Solar plexus chakra jewelry is often used to assist with mental problems, spirituality, and all physical and mental development maters.

Syadisthana or the sacral chakra is the sixth chakra. It is situated inside the body's sacrum. It is known that the ovaries and other sexual organs and the menstrual cycle are directly linked. A lotus with six petals, along with the beautiful orange shade, symbolizes it. The jewelry of the Sacral Chakra is used to assist with fertility issues. It can also be used to assist with religious zeal and imagination.

Last but not least, you've got the Muladhara (base chakra). Instinct, safety, and basic human survival are thought to be directly related. It is located near the vagina at the pelvis base. While no endocrine organ is within its source, gonads and adrenal medulla are thought to be directly related. Which is responsible for our response to battle or flight. The Muladhara is depicted by a four-petalled lotus and adorned with the vibrant red hues. The jewelry of the Muladhara chakra is often used to assist with attraction, mental stability, sensuality, and a sense of security.

CHAPTER SIX:

The Interconnection of Seven Chakras and Seven Colors

Throughout our life, the seven chakras and the seven colors play an important role. Increasing color has special healing power and is demonstrated in the seven chakras of meditation.

What is meditation?

7 Chakras, what are they?

How're our life-related colors?

What is relaxation exactly?

This comes from two Latin words: mediating (exercising the brain, thought, calming nature), modern means healing. The derivation from Sanskrit Medha means Wisdom. It is mindfulness to observe our breath with consciousness and to do anything with the knowledge. We understand the structure and function of our mind by communicating with a particular practice of meditation.

It is the reflective, deep silence state which happens when the mind is calm and still and fully conscious. It is the means of changing the mind; it encourages and creates in our life focus and clarity, emotional positivity. It is a way of living; it is the end of the process of thought.

What is Chakra Seven?

Chakra is the Sanskrit word meaning "the wheel." There are seven big chakras in the spinal column and cross the body's ring. Every Chakra has the number of correct qualities that suit the energy improvement from the base level stuff, self-identity located at the first Chakra to the higher spirit-level knowledge of being at our Crown. These energy centers reflect our highest level of broken, prism-like incorporation into a color spectrum. The essence of the unified field of creativity is by mastering each chakra. We rearrange our desperate part into a full self-awareness radiant light.

That chakra is connected with a specific part of the body and a certain organ that provides the power that it needs to function on a mental and spiritual level. Our state of health and wellbeing is dictated by the transparency and flow of energy into our chakra.

The Seven Chakras and Seven Colors Each center has its central purpose of maintaining our energy balance; by studying the energetic and physical being, we can create wellness, emotional stability, and spiritual bliss.

The first stage is known as the spinal cord-based Root Chakra (Muladhara), marked by red color, the seat of physical strength, and the essential desire to live. It controls the processes that keep the body alive. It is the chakra that has innocence as its main feature.

The Second Degree is classified slightly below Naval as the Sacral Chakra (Swadhisthana), shown in the color of Orange. This energy is the core of all kinds of relationship formation. It is where we develop an internal sense of self and the outer sense of other people, ego, sexuality, and family, and establish how we function as power. Certain people's feeling is experienced directly through the manipulation of the energy of this chakra.

The third tier is called the Solar Plexus Chakra (Manipura), which is also just above the Naval. The position where the energy is transmitted is situated in the middle of the body. It is the core of emotional and personal energy that is unrefined. It is the core that brings us a sense of total contentment and satisfaction. The imagination is motivated by the willpower.

The fourth level at the center of the chest is the Heart Chakra (Anahata), indicated by the Green shade. The source of true unconditional affection, spiritual growth, empathy, love, and devotion. It is the bridge that links our being's lower and higher energies and the place where our Soul, our real, free and independent self, resides.

The fifth stage is known as the Throat Chakra (Vishuddha) at the chest, marked by the color Blue. This is where the inner voice of one's reality is revealed, the source of communication, self-expression, and imagination. It is the chakra of communication and pure friendship with others, one's being's interconnectivity.

The sixth stage is known as the third eye chakra (Ajna) in the middle of the forehead and is marked by the color of the indigo. It is here that we imagine the seat of insight and direct divine vision through our "fourth sight" or intuitive awareness. A third-eye opening leads to "spiritual awakening." It is the chakra of compassion and forgiveness.

The Seventh and final level is Crown Chakra (Shasarar) it is at the top of the head indicates Violet color, this tier reflects the highest level of consciousness and liberation, it is the connective center of the soul, and this center combines all the chakra with their respective qualities. Mastering our being's lower vibration dimension we live in the full awareness that we are living a human existence as a divine being.

How is the color associated with our lives?

All the colors in our life are very necessary; they have important characteristics that signify a powerful significance in our life.

The vibrant Red color is the "Great Energizer" and "The Vitality Dad." Red is moist, critical, and warming, removing or opening all clogs, releasing rigidity and constraints. It is the color of strength, bravery, and faith in oneself.

Orange is a mixture of red and yellow, mixing physical energy with mental intelligence, resulting in a transition between lower physical reaction and higher mental response; it is often referred to as the "Intelligence Ray." It is the color of moist, loving and non-constructive, assimilating new ideas and stimulating cognitive awareness, as well as helping deal with inappropriate sexual expression.

Yellow helps to improve the nerve and brain, it helps to promote mental energy and a higher mindset. Yellow is

"Worth its Gold weight." It can be used for liver, liver and intestinal disorders, helps the skin pores and helps scarred tissue repair itself, has a very enriching effect on the mind and brain. Yellow color, by our cognitive selves, binds us.

The next color in the line is Green, our Mother Nature and Earth's color and natural healing. The most organic and environmentally friendly color has an exciting effect as well as a calming effect. Green is combining color, peace, nurture, neutrality, and non-resistance. Green vegetables have magical effects on our appetite, they provide all the nutrients needed to build our body. Our body feels comfortable by seeing the greenery and relaxes our bodies, nerves, and views.

Blue is known for its calming qualities, one of the world's largest antiseptics is "the Blue-ray." One of the psychologically soothing colors, it has a specific effect on the nervous system and provides great stimulation, suitable for children with sleep problems and hyperactivity. It also leads us to holistic ideas and strengthens interaction and expression by giving us insight and clarity. Blue is also the vast ocean's shade.

Indigo is the liberating and purifying agent color that helps the flow of blood and mental problems. It is also a light that the spirits use to help the medium join. It is also described as the solar system's light. It is particularly used to cure diseases such as cataracts, glaucoma, and other problems with the eyes. This binds the brow chakra (third eye) which activates the pineal glands and stimulates them. This affects both physical and spiritual experiences, and coping with the aspects of eye and ear issues can be of great help. Indigo is known as the Holy Spirit's light.

Violet is the Divine Spirit's light, it works on at the spirit level. Generally speaking, this color is not used for physical conditions, but some experts believe it offers nourishment to the upper brain cells and has a link to the crown chakra. We are linked by violet energy with our spiritual guidance, wisdom and inner strength.

White is the color of the awakening spirit, the purity light; it is the Divine Light shade. When we learn about the people surrounded by the "White Healing and

Security Light." It is the most physical location above the crown.

Chakra Balancing With Healing Stones

Each of us has a very complex energy body system. - aura has an extremely definite and very individualistic boundary, but at the same time one must also be mindful that each energy body is real energy, so it can not remain isolated. Their energies are constantly exposed to so many other energy bodies as a result of which they are vulnerable to blurry, open, and off sync chakras. It's quick to heal the chakra and can be extremely beneficial. Stone use facilitates and intensifies the process of healing and alignment.

There are several stones appropriate for each chakra. Below are the 4 most common crystals used for the respective chakras: Root Chakra-Red-Grounding-Spine base (stones can also be put at the feet)

1. Bloodstone-Helps relieve anxieties that can cause the body to unbalance Promotes detoxification while improving the kidneys, liver and spleen

2. Agate-Increase self-esteem, improve physical and emotional protection to reduce negativity

3. Smoky Quartz-An excellent grounding crystal that lets one concentrate on the present Effective in dissolving negative energy and emotional blockages

4. Tiger's Eye-Encourages confidence and patience Sacred

Chakra-Orange-Joy-just below the button of the belly

1. Citrine-Helps emotional maturity growth Effective during times of emotional instability

2. Carnelian-Helps remove sorrow from the emotional self Promotes the physical energy needed to act in emotionally challenging circumstances

3. Moonstone-Helps to strengthen the feminine side Calms feelings to look more critically at a situation

4. Rutilated Quartz-This stone is important for all chakras of meditation, healing, and spiritual development Helps to stabilize relationships and emotional imbalances Solar Plexus— Yellow— Development, Physical Health, and Creativity —

Naval and sternum base

1. Calcite-(golden or yellow) Helpful with pancreatic, kidney and spleen dysfunctions Helpful with kick-starting the Solar Plexus after clearing

2. Malachite-Helps to tie the Solar Plexus to the Heart Chakra to promote the empathy necessary to prevent the misplacement of personal power

3. Sunstone-Thought to bring good luck Good to relieve pain in the stomach and ulcers

4. Yellow Citrine-Helps one to gain access to his power and increases self-confidence Good to resolve addictions and digestive problems Heart Chakra-

Green-Compassion and Unconditional Love-Chest Center

1. Rose Quartz-Helps one becomes more open to joy Heals emotional wounds

2. Green Jade-Speaker to provide reassurance and support for vulnerable people

3. Aventurine Quartz-Depression Great Encourages life excitement

4. Watermelon Tourmaline-Known as Heart Chakra's' super activator' and interacts with Throat Chakra-Blue-Communication-Throat

1. Lapis Lazuli-Increase knowledge and intellectual capacity Improve the mental clarity required to communicate effectively with others

2. Celestite-Can help with clairaudience and recall of dreams Mental clarity

3. Saying to help you find your true path Effective in creative endeavors

4. Sodalite-Fosters objectivity and new perspectives, offering a balance between minds of consciousness and unconsciousness Clarity on how to go forward in life Third Eye Chakra-Indigo-Intuition and Intelligence-Just above and between eyes

1.Calcite-Aid to boost third eye

2 energies. Purple Fluorite-Brings logic and intuition together Improve the ability to concentrate and eradicate false perceptions

3. Azurite-Effective if blocked or underused

4 to activate the Third Eye. Amethyst-A helpful and defensive force that produces a calming influence when one is overwhelmed by intellectual and emotional chaos of Crown Chakra-Violet-Spirituality and selflessness-Top of Head

1. Clear Quartz-An An' all-purpose' healing crystal that can enhance, concentrate and transform energy Believed to help Kundalini energy movement attain spiritual power

2. 2 realizations. Herkimer Diamond-Bring's positive balance throughout the body Great antidepressant Promotes a desire to be more than

3. Amethyst-Creates a sense of peace and contentment

4. 4 in letting go and trusting. Diamond-Saying to encourage faith and keep negativity away Symbol of perfection; helping us to step towards our highest spiritual potential Lie on your back, holding arms uncrossed on your sides and legs. Place the stones on the correct chakras from the Root Chakra to the Crown Chakra. Hold it on your body until it slows down your brain. It is important to reach one of the slower brain wave states to make your body respond to the healing process, but not to fall asleep. If you are one who frequently meditates or has some knowledge of doing so, meditates for at least 15 minutes with the stones on your chakras. If meditation is new

to you, you can find it very easy for the beginner to listen to a CD with a guided meditation.

Make sure to clean your stones once you've done your meditation with the rocks. You are going to absorb unnecessary energy and need washing.

To do this, there is more than one process, but the easiest way is to use sea salt. Salt can be mixed or dried with salt. Combine a tablespoon of sea salt in a glass of cold water ceramic mug when using saltwater. Do not use containers made of metal or plastic. In the water, position the stones and allow them to soak overnight. Place the sea salt in a glass or non-plastic bowl to use dry salt and cover the crystals with the points in the salt facing down. Let's go overnight again. A stone can sometimes take longer to clear, particularly if used in deep, intense healing. If that's the case, save the sea salt for another day or two. It is possible to use the dry sea salt process to remove gemstone necklaces. Make sure you only use salt from the ocean, not salt from the bowl. Aluminum and other contaminants are found in table salt.

Another easy way is to use some white sage and burn it until your sage gets a good strong smoke. For at least one minute, preferably three or four minutes, keep the stone in this smoke.

The Root Chakra Issues on self-coaching

The first or root Chakra (Sanskrit Muladhara) is located at the base of the spine, at the perineum, the area between the genitals and the rectum.

This chakra has to do with family issues, community issues, and tribal issues. It is our life force's home and it maintains our physical health and vitality as it is the nucleus that binds us to the Earth's sustaining energy and physical truth. It is also the source of the masculine power within us (whether we are a man or a woman) and it provides the seeds of our full potential. Our first chakra resonates on the color spectrum with the color red in the auric region and the harmonic scale with the C note.

The primary function of the root chakra is to focus our attention on what we need to survive and thrive in life daily. It is through this chakra that we encounter the world for the first time as we are still in the womb and in the first year of our lives. If we grow up with enough attention, affection and loving emotions, with parents who felt safe and rooted in confidence themselves, it's most likely that our first chakra will evolve healthily and we'll feel safe and worthy of love as a consequence. Nevertheless, when our external circumstances (past or present) become dysfunctional, our mental growth is destabilized and our consciousness is fogged with the central conviction that the universe is a precarious place to fight for survival. This conviction will then serve as a promise which fulfills itself, attracting in our life circumstances that justify its presence. All changes including moving, divorcing, having a baby, mourning, natural disasters, fighting, physical abuse, and financial hardship can also build a first chakra level imbalance.

There may be a lack of physical endurance but also psychological strength in the first chakra problems. There are fear and depression instead of feeling safe and secure in the world. Perhaps you may be out of control with overemphasis attachment to material possessions, security or sensual thrills.

The alignment of this chakra is therefore essential to developing with a fundamental sense of security and stability in life. This in effect empowers us to trust life itself, because we view the world as a place where food, shelter, and protection can be adequately provided.

There are many shadow facets of the first chakra, most of which are based on fear of lack, which, as we have already described, creates conditions of scarcity and uncertainty, thus reinforcing beliefs focused on lack and fear of lack. It's a vicious circle, as you see.

Similar shadows aspects of the first chakra imbalance are fear, depression, restlessness, disorganization, anxiety about not being enough, feelings of indignity, feelings of abandonment, weak boundaries, lack of consideration for others, lack of confidence in others, rigidity, defensiveness, distrust...

On the physical side: overweight and extremely underweight, eating disorders, bone and teeth disorders, spine issues, intestines, arms, feet, knees.

Self-Application: While there are many facets of this first chakra that we could discuss, we will concentrate on the idea of limiting beliefs for this course: Key point 1: Limiting belief is a conviction that you have about yourself or some aspect of your life that prevents you from being the person you could be-or from doing or doing things you could have or do if you didn't. These may be statements that our parents or teachers taught us and we adopted them as our own, without really questioning whether they are true to us.

Limiting principles often come from our fears-they can be used as a means of self-protection to stop our fears from being confronted. The problem with restricting beliefs is that they are self-reinforcing: you build what you feel is possible for you, and you reproduce the same results in your life over and over.

Here are some examples of restricting values when they apply to the first issues of the chakra: "It's hard to make a living"-When we look at life from a difficult place, we create more difficult situations in our life, and "It's hard to make a living" would continue to be true for us.

"Successful people are arrogant"-this idea is inconsistent with success and will discourage us from attracting them to us.

"Rich people are not religious"-This is a common belief, particularly in so-called spiritual circles, where wealth is often associated with hypocrisy and authenticity. While this may be true in some cases, judging people about how much money they have is per se rather restricting and will ultimately work against any deliberate effort to earn some money.

Key point 2: The risk with these restricting convictions is that they are most often subconscious and work secretly in our lives, often as saboteurs of our most aware projects.

This week's fieldwork: 1. Begin analyzing your thoughts this week and know that restricting values can continue to come up for you all day long. Listen to your internal dialog and be conscious if you think about someone or a situation.

To put it another way, catch yourself thinking, start to become more mindful of the words you use in your vocabulary.

What are the convictions below these words and thoughts?

Which theories do you make of your life that keep you stuck repeating the past?

Throughout the day, what are you doing that recreates the same negativity over and over?

Describe and jot down every day one belief about security, money or property in general.

2. To do this exercise, find a quiet moment at night or in the morning: sit comfortably on a chair or cross-legged

with your spine straight on the ground. Hold a sheet of paper by your hand-and a pad-as you later need it.

Begin breathing from your spine's root and concentrate on that region while taking deep breaths into it. Rest your hands and think or visualize the color red on your abdomen.

First Exercise: Ask yourself: from my root chakra what do I broadcast to the universe?

Do I feel that there is plenty of everything for all, or am I stuck in a mindset of scarcity where things are such that I can just have enough to get by?

How secure do I make it sound in the world? Do I have faith in new people and situations or do I find it hard to get out of my comfort zone?

Rest in your root chakra's power for a moment and think about one belief that you found during the day.

Ask yourself, is this true?

Is that true?

Live sufficiently long with these two questions. You ought to come to a point where you are beginning to doubt that what you believed is true.

Now, ask yourself: when I think this question, how do I react?

Remember what you're doing, stick with the emotions. Allow them to emerge when negative feelings occur, do not try to push them back.

Finally, ask yourself: Without this thought, who would I be?

Stay with the problem. Let your whole being penetrate it.

(These questions are taken from Byron Katie's Turnaround process, to learn more about the wonderful work of Byron Katie, go to thework.com) Go back to your bed, and as you keep taking deep long red breaths into the root of your spine, think about what you've managed to do so far.

Second exercise: Be mindful of what you have already achieved, gained and accomplished so far in your life, and relax in the knowledge that you have succeeded in delivering these things for yourself, and there is no particular reason to believe that this will ever change.

Continue to think about more things you've been able to realize and provide for yourself.

Feel like this realization makes you feel a little more comfortable.

Stay in this sense of trust and honesty.

Just a few more minutes, breathe it.

It no longer becomes such a scary place to be when you relax and trust the world to take care of you.

Everything you can be, do and have is planted in the root chakra, and when your actions and your sense of being embedded in this core of energy they can be fed by your life force rather than by stress, business or concern. All you need to do is allow yourself to open your consciousness to this core of energy and begin to explore your full potential.

I urge you starting today to integrate these activities into your life. Be proactive; commit to starting this self-discovery journey. You're not going to regret that. Hold your thoughts paper daily...

The more you put into these workouts, the more you benefit from them. You will begin to feel subtle changes in your sense of being as you go on. You that feel more grounded, more present, and more mindful of the relation between your beliefs and truth.

CHAPTER SEVEN:
Power of the Heart Chakra

Many are pursuing healing techniques, some of which are based on Eastern (not necessarily geographic) traditions such as yoga, chi quoting, and tai chi. Spiritual practices and beliefs exist all over the world, with the same message in different cultures and belief systems. If we could just sit still and listen to our inner voices, our internal encouragement, we can heal ourselves, to experience the interconnectedness with the world.

Heart culture is developing. There is coming age of imagination and empathy. In this new age, the heart plays a leading role... Healthy Heart Meditation Healing with the chakras to release the toxic effects of daily stress is believed to be popularized by the New Age Movement. These energy centers can help bring harmony to life, feel more positive and help neutralize create in our lives. Via meditation, accessing and calming the chakras can activate the energy centers. And what's that chakra?

Chakra The word chakra derives from a Sanskrit word meaning circle, a wheel that spins. Many who deal with chakras, with their specific color, can see each primary chakra as a spinning vortex. Chakras activate specific energy system areas. There are many chakra points in the human body, but the emphasis is on the seven primary chakras for healing and soothing purposes. The seven chakras are situated in ascending order along the spinal column from the base of the spine to the top of the head.

The Chakra of the Heart The heart is the location of our passions. It's fragile and easy to break, but incredibly durable. There's no point trying to deceive the soul. For its existence, it depends on our sincerity... The heart is the source of love, a network of human energy. Is love curing everything? Who didn't feel the agony of a broken heart, sadness, and remorse, the crippling impact of loss, emotional problems, alienation, rejection, separation— just to name a few in a long list of hurtful situations? To dry a damaged heart's tears, it needs more than physical healing. When ignored, heart pain will affect the soul, it will disrupt strength, brain, body, and spirit. Medical attention is not enough to treat heart problems more often than not.

Believe it or not, all of us are connected to the Almighty. We have the gift of perception, feeling, awareness. To see us through the bad times and appreciate the good times, we just need to know how to tap into these talents. Is the blind faith sufficient? Not every one of us is willing to believe, let alone open our minds to find a deeper connection with the Divine.

In the middle of your chest is the heart chakra, in Sanskrit, it is Anahata Chakra, which means unstuck. It is associated with the spiritual and physical self. It's our external bodies ' midpoint. It lies between the three lower chakras that hold us in the physical realm going. There are three upper chakras above the heart chakras that allow us to flourish in the spiritual realm where our emotions, imagination, intuition, and creativity can be realized.

Those who support chakra healing and calming the key chakra energies claim that this brings about the healing of pain, opens the intuitive ability with which we are born, calms the mind and paves the way for inner peace. We learn to let life flow, to be more appreciative of the endless blessings to which we are blind. We come to realize that our waking hours need not be consumed by concerns and fears, thereby tormenting the unconscious.

Through the chakra of the heart, we understand and embrace the value of unconditional love that is available to us all. This comprises the other six major chakras as the heart chakra grows, putting the physical and the divine self into harmony, thus bringing life into balance. Meditating on the chakra of the heart extends the sense of emotions, words, and deeds— it brings us into the real meaning of love— a love that is infinite and unconditional.

The heart chakra radiates energy that allows us to live lives that are rich and satisfying. It is a guiding force that binds the physical and spiritual worlds that help us stop being self-centered, un-careful, feeling like a victim and other negative attributes. The heart chakra is the center where we attract abundance to our lives so we can share it with others. We share a world beyond ourselves, we step beyond our physical world's obvious limits, be more conscious and aware that we are all linked. That's said more quickly than done.

Multiple forms of meditation exist. Working with the chakras together with visualization is a meditative operation. On the Internet, sites are offering good meditative practice on the chakra of the heart. Meditation is a very personal preference.

Manifesting Through the Chakras

It wasn't too long ago that we were unaware of issues like chakras in human history. The topic is nearly popular today. They're energy centers or vortexes that exist within and around your physical body in the off chance you've never heard of chakras.

Even if you're not familiar with chakras, your power has already been felt. You feel the energy of the fourth chakra-the heart chakra-when you feel a sense of love coming from your heart. You experience a direct hit to your third chakra, your core of personal power if you feel like someone knocked the wind out of you by breaking one of your boundaries.

All over your body, you have chakras and even outside your skin. Such chakras outside your body, like your aura, are in your other energy fields or spirit bodies.

This section deals only with the seven big chakras in your physical body. Such seven chakras are aligned horizontally from the top of your head to the base of your torso in the middle of your body.

Both chakras ' opening faces away from the physical body. The fulcrum of the seven main chakras is linked to the central pipe of the power of life force, or prana, which runs vertically through the human body's head and torso, as in the right image.

Chakras function as knowledge receptors and transmitters, making them important creative devices- from inspiration to realization.

The process of creating through the chakras starts at the Crown Chakra and flows as follows through the other six: the Seventh Chakra: commonly known as the Crown Chakra, is located at the top of your head, or crown. It is where you are guided by your guides, angels, the Higher Self, and other sacred sources of higher knowledge for your plan or task.

Your Third Eye Chakra is where you perceive your inspiration's visual form and "see" it with your inner vision.

The Fifth Chakra: This chakra is in the middle of your throat where you turn thought and sight into words. This is the first manifestation of the inspiration you have received through your crown chakra on the physical plane.

The Fourth Chakra: Sometimes called the "heart chakra," it is found in your heart's area and is associated with the feeling of love. Your chakra of the heart is where you feel your inspiration's love and passion.

The Third Chakra: This is your private will's nucleus. It is situated in your solar plexus and is where, as you step into motion, you produce and concentrate the force of your energy or drive.

The Second Chakra: Also called the Sacral Chakra, it is found in your lower abdomen, a few inches below your belly button. This chakra is associated with family, friends, and culture. Your sacral chakra is where you share your inspiration with other people. The First Chakra: commonly called the Root Chakra.

The Chakras Are Organs of the Ethereal Body

The chakras are the ethereal body's organs that work in harmony with the physical organs to allow the physical bodies to develop into beautiful forms through which the Creator's spirit may enter and communicate.

The chakras are power centers, vibrating atoms storehouses, the first life stirrings in the universe. At the start, it was simply the wind that played around and raised sand grains that had crumbled off the smooth rock surfaces and put them near the water on the ground. This triggered a chemical reaction between the soil's minerals and the water's algae. This gave birth to the Kingdom of Botany and provided a method for embedding this power.

The root chakra, the first chakra, was the first energy package to be expressed in the physical matter in a manifested form. The Botanical Kingdom evolved into the one cell amoeba by decaying and rotting material. The only chakra in these early life forms was the root chakra or kundalini. The sum being for life-giving properties and energies were based in that kundalini. It was the core of the vibrating atoms and was needed when the animals used their tail for means of locomotion and defense in those early forms of life.

In the animals to proceed into the human world, the root chakra was not required, as they would no longer need the tail. The tail was sealed over this chakra and eventually disappeared from the man. In the second chakra, the sacral plexus, the bundle of energy was then implanted to ensure the race's existence. The second chakra, the sacral plexus, was the only one functioning in the "caveman." It is the core of life, human instinct such as feeding, sleeping, and procreation.

The third chakra, the solar plexus, was slowly established. In the early days of Lemuria, it was only a stage before the third center was established by Lemuria called Lamanai. This third focus, which was the awareness of the thoughts of others, formed as the primitive man felt a definite need to interact with his kind to distinguish between himself and the animals. It was a very slow process as the second chakra's power was not turned off. It had to be protected, so this third chakra or energy center had to grow and create and evolve from scratch.

The introduction of the heart chakra at the same time that these basic creatures formed a conscience, a need to feel responsible for their actions against others, followed this phase more rapidly. This heart chakra was a rapidly developing one, as preventing the animal/men from killing each other was urgently needed. Thus the animal following his impulses started to have feelings and emotions to deal with. Due to the heavy activity of the second and fourth centers, the third center, the solar plexus, was not intentionally shut down but fell into disuse.

Thus the animal types had formed into an upright, almost tailless shape which began to feel the difference between them and the animals that remained on all four. We started letting us know what the basic grunts and sign language meant. Sensing the thoughts of others, this ESP, so to speak, is beginning to fade, and requiring a means to communicate, the throat chakra drew the bundle of energy from the solar plexus to the throat, and the fifth chakra was formed. The grunts were distinctive, smart sounds that quickly developed into a language.

The next chakra, the third eye, evolved partly because of the deviousness and ingenuity and deceit of man, and partly because of the solar plexus being disused. They used their imagination to imagine what the other was thinking, try to second-guess the other, play games, makeup stories, tell fairy tales, and get the other to react to games and daydreams when they wanted to know what others were thinking so they could manipulate them or beat them while inventing something. This took too much drastic action when this was carried out and the Atlantean civilization was ruined.

Civilization was initiated by reforming the chakra structure, but not straight down to the one cell again. There was still no need to use the first chakra and at this time it was fully sealed. The second was still in use, the third was restored, the fourth more isolated from the second, more independently working from the second's intuition. The fifth was left as it was, the sixth shut down, sealed off, and added the spot for the seventh chakra. The energy from the sixth center was sent to the seventh center, but it was still sealed off until it was needed and healthy to bring to humanity.

The targets are set by the three lower chakras. The root chakra gives the push, the ability to live, the power to step forward. The second chakra, the sacral plexus, gives you the imagination to create your own life, and the third chakra gives you the ability to communicate psychically with other realms and men. In the three higher realms, the throat chakra gives you the ability to connect with other kingdoms and share your ambitions and imagination. The sixth chakra, the third eye allows you to envision imagination, and the crown chakra enables you to connect with the higher realms. The fourth chakra, the chakra of the heart, functions as a conduit that enables all the other chakras to work together.

The heart chakra turns the animal kingdom's instinctual actions into being a human being's physical development. Without these transformative powers, mankind would not have gone so far as to act as vessels of speech for the spirits to join. The three lower kingdoms derive from the physical nature that went before you. The three higher kingdoms allow you to access a spiritual nature that went before you. Both of these are used to shape your heart chakra universe.

CHAPTER EIGHT:
Crystal-Healing the Chakras

Who truly understands the chakras among us? Much is still undiscovered for all that we know about these seven spinal energy levels.

The chakras appear as light spinning wheels, according to ancient texts. Yes, the word chakra is wheel Sanskrit. Chakras obtain and emit energy that, depending on the health of this energy, can be either negative or positive. You will discover variations in the needs of each chakra during the healing process. You don't have to fear this challenge. Think of your chakras as a garden that needs specialized care for each flower. Many chakras will need less focus, while others will need less attention. The commitment to this self-examination makes it as difficult as it is satisfying to heal the chakras.

You can change the guidelines below to suit your needs. Be alert not to the size or appearance when selecting stones, but rather to your reaction when keeping them.

Some of these crystals may be uncommon, but in a mystical or rock shop, you are likely to find them. Although you may enjoy this introduction to chakra healing, with the guidance of a trained professional, it is best to undergo long-term care. Most skilled chakra healers are extremely intuitive in addition to being experienced. Their critical analysis will help you understand each imbalance's reasons. In and of itself, this can be soothing.

First Chakra: This is the chakra of the heart. It's at the spine's foundation or tailbone. The root chakra is part of the physical world. This chakra needs little attention if you feel grounded, safe, and rooted in the present. Others, however, are not so lucky. A blocked root chakra may cause you to forget the physical, become overly possessive and clingy. Conversely, you can feel alienated from your body and belongings if you're too transparent here. As a result, you can take advantage of your kindness.

Crystal Correction: Obsidian opens a blocked chakra. This gem offers a concentrated, calm outlook so that an appreciation of the temporary nature of possessions eliminates the desire to compulsively accumulate. Place a piece of obsidian on your genital area while lying on your back to repair cracks. When you relax more the strength of the stone will interact with your own, it will strengthen. Rose quartz is required for an abundantly open core. Soft pink quartz, while typically associated with the brain, helps us to embrace and enjoy ourselves, so we can protect ourselves by saying no.

2nd Chakra: The sacral chakra governs our sexual energy and creativity. To feel its position, you just need to click two inches below your navel. A happy sacral chakra's gift is expressivity and flair. A blockage may lead to new ideas being resisted

Crystal Correction: Carnelian: this quartz variety is perfect for the sacred area to be opened. Although it can be found in many colors, the cautious is granted courage by the stimulating qualities of red or orange. This helps us to fulfill our goals without blocking our path with fear-based hallucinations. If this chakra is too accessible, you may need lapis Luiz, on the other hand. In ancient Egypt and Babylon, this iconic light blue stone was highly valued. Today, to help us behave carefully, we can use its moderating powers. Scott Cunningham writes in Crystal, Gems & Metal Magic: "Simply touching the body with this stone will enhance your psychological, physical, spiritual, metaphysical and emotional health." Rest this stone as long as needed for maximum benefits to the 2nd chakra.

3rd Chakra: This is your solar plexus, also known as the center of power. A pool of unexplored will and bravery remains here. We know our potential and are inspired to fulfill it when this chakra is safe. We can experience "butterflies in our belly" or suffer from other stomach woes when blocked. A blocked core of control makes us feel weak and helpless. When this energy core is too small, the opposite problem occurs.

Golden Beryl is a small, lemon yellow stone that guides will and enhances trust. It is therefore good for blockages of the 3rd chakra. Placing this two-inch stone above your navel will free your power center and help you achieve your goals. Green jade is for those who are confused by this chakra. The calming stone helps to gently and harmlessly guide our emotions, through destructive thoughts to others.

4th Chakra: This is the chakra of the heart and is self-explanatory in its context. This is the spiritual development, devotion, strength, and high ideals divine domain. A stuffy chakra of the heart makes us excessively critical of both ourselves and others. We find it hard to open ourselves up to possibilities of love and friendship in this situation. When, on the other hand, our heart is too big, we can try to do the impossible by trying to carry the world's weight.

Crystal Correction: The green jasper put on the heart allows us to feel safe enough to open up and reveal ourselves. It promotes contact that is frank and cheerful. Seek peridot for a soul without boundaries. Also this soft, pastel green stone charges us by calming us down. Peridot helps us to be sweet, but not sacrificial.

5th Chakra: The chakra of the throat allows us to connect through words as well as physical. It's found at the throat bottom. We speak honestly and freely when this chakra is healthy. The deceit is subtle if we are blocked here. We can, for example, leave out details. Additionally, we speak too much and without forethought when this chakra is expanded. This is commonly referred to as the condition of "foot in the face."

Crystal Correction: Sodalite; a stunning navy stone that assists with the chakra of the heart. It brings us confidence and clarity in this stone. We can sound it with confidence knowing our facts. Those with an extensive 5th chakra, on the other hand, need to sound their reality quieter. Amber is helpful in that capacity. This rock is soulful deeply. Kevin Sullivan explains in The Crystal Handbook that "Amber represented the resting place of the spirit or spirits thought to animate the rock in Viennese mystic literature." Fossilized, multimillion-year-old tree sap, amber provides us with early earth's natural knowledge.

6th Chakra: This power core is regarded to many as the 3rd eye between the brows. This chakra gives us the ability to see beyond appearances if in harmony, exposing our inherent psychic abilities. But, when it is blocked, we restrict ourselves to evidence that has not been investigated. It leads to rigid thinking and happiness that has been disrupted. Nonetheless, we may be separated from the physical world if we're too transparent here. The inability to close the psychic eye fills with a confounding feeling of unreality when it suits. Equilibrium is essential. We also have to wake up Crystal Correction when we dream: a moonstone put on the 6th chakra will clear up the problems that blind our instincts and open the mind to the unseen. This encourages personal growth because moonstone is linked to cycles of transition. It allows us to adapt to motion, to accept spontaneity and to release rigidity. Blue lace agate is needed with an overly open 3rd eye. A stunning, sky-blue stone sharpens our attention, removing the emotional diversion clutter.

Chakra 7: Awesome! Words are not enough to convey the crown chakra's power. This chakra, situated at the top center of your face, offers the possibility of enlightenment. Although balancing it will not make us a Buddha, it will certainly bring us to spiritual happiness heights and connect us with the meaning of our life. You're far from alone if you're stuck here. It's unusual to have a balanced crown chakra. To spiritual self-development, it is the blessing of tireless efforts. We may be uncertain about our profession if blocked and lack permanent, rapturous calm. We must first ensure the well-being of our previous chakras for maximum results in balancing this chakra. It is rarely a problem to have this chakra too open unless you hate happiness and harmony. We're all living among the disillusioned. We have to be able to communicate with the cynic as well as the sorry. Otherwise, in our minds, we are stuck. It can get pretty lonely as safe as this place is.

Crystal Correction: Clear quartz for all chakras is a trustworthy healer, but it is particularly useful in opening the closed crown. The chosen crystal should be small enough to sit on the top of your head due to the location of the seventh chakras. The stone offers clarity of purpose and allows us in everyday events to see the broader meaning. In doing so, it helps us to understand universal truths and to live by harmony. Hematite is soothing for those with the excessively open crown chakra. It's grounding as well. The dark and strong stone will help us fulfill our own and otherworldly needs by drawing attention to the practical realities of life.

Major Chakara

Citizens everywhere are realizing the value and usefulness of energy healing, whether they agree that all is energy or not because we are going into a time of increased awareness, tolerance, and capabilities with the increasing vibration of citizens as a whole.

My vision is to see the earth where everyone knows the value of a balanced, energetic body, and regular exercises of chakra become the norm. Such spiritual chakras help regulate the internal organs and glands, thereby keeping you physically healthier. These also help regulate one's feelings, which is why these help you stay mentally and emotionally healthier. The chakras being in a balanced state of thus helping to bring peace to your whole being, promoting a genuinely holistic state of health.

We as a race of people nowadays MUST learn to #1 Be conscious of their current chakras #2 continue to keep the seven major chakras safe. Keeping the seven major centers healthy is necessary because we are gradually moving into another dimension of existence and to do so our bodies must reach a higher vibration and frequency.

The seven they are now using must be in a healthy state of being for these five to awaken.

A summary of the seven major chakras is as follows: ROOT CHAKRA 1st middle, around the sex organs between the thighs. Gland: Gland of adrenals. Suprarenal glands (cortisone, adrenaline, noradrenaline) are red and black in their primary color. Main focus: SURVIVAL, PHYSICAL NEEDS, GROUNDEDNESS. The keywords here are "To Be To Have." Scents are Vetiver and Sandalwood. An open and stable root chakra helps solid structural elements of the physical body to be grounded (earth and nature support); spinal column, adrenals, kidneys, arms, ribs, teeth, feet, knees, lower back, hair, large intestine, pelvic area, and eliminatory process smooth operations. The root chakra binds everything to the ground, caring for the legs and feet, sciatic nerve, blood pressure. Allergic reactions are also associated with the root chakra.

When you have a good root chakra, you stand firmly on the ground with both feet. It relates to one's willingness to live, sense of security, instincts and basic interaction, issues related to food, clothes, shelter-practical things, self-preservation, stamina, rhythm and nature relation...

2nd section of SACRAL CHAKRA; lower to navel abdomen. Gland: Gonads, you know. Testicles and ovaries (testosterone and estrogen) The color is red. Main focus: VITALITY, DESIRE, SELF-WORTH, CREATIVITY. "Feeling, Wanting." Scents: Patchouli, Ylang Ylang. A well-developed sacral chakra protects the reproductive system's health; testicles, penis, ovaries and uterus, duodenum, ileum, cecum, lower vertebrae, small intestine, pelvis, urinary tract, bladder. Impotence is also avoided and menstrual pain is reduced. A strong sacral chakra assimilates meat, detoxifies the skin, enhances the immune system. Energy, procreation, fertility and healthy sexual activity, imagination, a love of living, resilience, harmonious relationships and working with others, compassion, surrender, motion, giving and receiving, all rely on a balanced sacral chakra...

Tweak Your Health and Happiness with Chakras

1. Root chakra (base of your spine, arms, blood, bones)-here we all feel rooted, protected and supported. It is our desire for survival, our ability to feel at home in our bodies, our bond with our immediate family. Think of the fundamentals: nutrition, shelter, money. Many related physical health problems include eating disorders, asthma, autoimmune disorders, and cancer of the rectum.

Tweaking advice for the root chakra: did a family member have unfinished business? Write them a letter, send it to yourself (not to them unless you know that the letter will do better than harm), read it, and burn it.
Get "grounded," plant a garden, take a walk, walk in the grass barefoot.
Eat veggies from the root and add more animal protein to your diet. So thank you for supporting you to the pets, crops, and people who grow / farm.
2. Sacred chakra (navel area, reproductive organs, liver, bladder, lower back)-The the second chakra is about

gender and imagination, personal ethics and morals, and actively engaging with others outside our family unit. Several related physical health conditions include lower back pain, reproductive organ disorders, cancer of the bladder, complications with pregnancy, and kidney disease.

Tweaking tips for the sacral chakra: think of your strength, gender, and money relationship. Are you somewhat over-controlled? Or are you innocent, disgraceful? Look for the balance.

Build a board of vision of what you want.

Prepare a meal with your family and share it.

Always interact with your food's flavors and texture.

Allow a sensual feeling of feeding.

3. Solar plexus (liver, digestion, pancreas, gallbladder and adrenals)—This is all about our self-worth, self-confidence, self-care, and how we see each other. Were you worried that you will fail? This is a common weakness of the third chakra. Anemia, ulcers, hypertension, digestive problems, and liver disease are some of the physical health issues linked to the solar plexus.

For the third chakra, tweaking tips: chew carefully. Chew well your food.

Take a long bath or construct a soothing routine before bedtime.

Prepare a meal with your family and share it.

Talk of yourself and remember who you are.

4. Heart chakra (circulatory system, heart, lungs)-love, unconditional love, empathy, compassion, tolerance for people who are different from us. Instead of cultivating self-love, an underactive heart chakra can manifest as feeling unloved, prejudice, and finding external esteem. Many heart chakra-related illnesses include heart disease, breathing problems, breast cancer, and upper back pain.

Tweaking tips for the chakra of the heart: lead by example.

Eat more acidic greens (watercress, kale, arugula, bok choy).

Hold a newspaper of appreciation.

5. Throat chakra (thyroid, ears, arms, neck)-This is where we are focusing on our desire to let go of material attachments and items that no longer serve us. That

chakra connects us to our soul and reflects our ability to effectively connect with others, our true voice. Thyroid problems, chronic sore throat, esophageal cancer, and pain in the shoulder and neck are some of the physical health issues associated with the throat chakra.

For the throat chakra, tweak tips: sing, participate in drama (the kind of play, not the kind of energy-sucking workplace), read.

Meditate when your breath is centered.

Show to others what you stand for.

6. Third eye (between eyebrows, pineal gland, eyes)- Have you ever had the moment of "wow!" This chakra has to do with intelligence, insight, and dreaming. Light and our circadian rhythm reflect it. Some mental disorders are expressed here: obsessive-compulsive behavior, distracted thought, often dependent on input from others, and poor self-awareness.

Sixth chakra tuning tips: tap your intuition. Switch off the appliances and sit down quietly. Listen to your voice inside. Practice that every day for 20 minutes.

Feed seasonally and locally, cooking with new herbs and spices.

Cut on alcohol and caffeine.

7. Crown chakra (top of the head, hypophyseal gland, cerebral cortex) — The seventh chakra is the most separated from the physical body and materials. It is our religion, our confidence in the power of God, and from where we derive faith and hope. The crown chakra's mental disorders include feeling lost in life, anxiety, psychosis, and suicidal thoughts without intent.

Balance Your Chakras With Self-Hypnosis

This approach is a step-by-step method that incorporates self-hypnosis with the concept of calming your chakras with some self-inner guidance. Now it's not important to know what your chakras are - in short, in Eastern medicine and philosophy they are known to be key energy points in your body. We are associated with certain colors that will be merged in your head into this technique.

I know that made me feel beautifully energized, refreshed and ultimately very well balanced.

Step One: Find a place where you will not be interrupted for a while, allowing you to close your eyelids. Think they melt and relax in your face when you close your eyelids and start sending relief across your body.

Build expectations; we all know how hypnotic it is to dream, don't we? Tell yourself that you will reach one of the most comfortable environments you've ever experienced in a few moments.

You can put yourself into self-hypnosis or use any effective mindfulness technique or relaxation method you know (if you don't know-how, go get my book). Take the breathing for a few moments and get interested in the moment. Note how you feel and think.

Step Two: Using your imagination, start to feel you're floating on a fluffy cloud, almost like a mist that's gentle, warm, and welcoming. It melds and molds itself to your body's exact contours, imagine you relax deeply into it and take enough time to develop the comfort.

Imagine the cloud is a beautiful red strawberry color, soft but solid.

Imagine the beautiful red mist enveloping the whole being soft. Notice that in a soft and gentle relaxation it bathes you.

Let that red mist pass your entire body, eliminating everything unwanted, leaving you in a warm, peaceful state. Picture the red color in every cell of your being. Let that red mist sink into the middle of your mind's very depths.

Spread the red into you, touch the tips of your toes all the way down to the tips of your fingers, and feel in harmony with this natural red color as your body becomes more balanced and alive.

Let your spine base dwell on the red mist. You might even believe that your spine is vibrating in unison with red and that the whole region of the lower back and spine is going into complete relaxation. You will produce many wonderful sensations when you are very engaged in doing this.

Dream and think that you are in harmony with nature and that all life is in harmony with you. Breathe in that red, gentle mist and now let a little, tiny red bird fly around you gently, covering your body in a warm, red, calming and soothing blanket.

If you're not a bird fan, you can, of course, imagine something else-angels or a loved one, or the blanket wraps around you without support. Do for yourself what suits you.

Step Three: Imagine floating on a light, almost peach-like orange color next up inside of your brain. Enable yourself to be in alignment with this orange (just like you were with the red) and there is an energy center vibrating with this orange color right around the region of your abdomen.

Allow this orange mist to add this gentle softness to your skin, this natural consciousness, and feel it almost like a sponge, absorbing and releasing anything you might want to let go of, soaking you in a calm mist of harmony, relaxation, and comfort. Sense and sense something unpleasant from all parts of your body being absorbed into the water.

Allow your body to penetrate this orange and give you peace and comfort, feel the freedom as you do this. Feel more and more soothing as this orange mist streams through and around every part of your abdomen. Then in whatever way you feel the best resonates with you, imagine a little orange ribbon gliding softly and gently bringing the mist around and through your skin, making your body perfectly relaxed and happy. Take enough time to make this a total pleasure.

Step Four: Imagine the soft color of lemon, perfect, lemon yellow right in the middle of your chest floating in your mind's eye.

Taking as long as you need to be in balance with this yellow color and the middle region of your body and the center of your neck is more and more soothing as you can imagine the area has an energy core that vibrates to the yellow color. Breathe in the soft yellow mist, let the warmth of that gentle softness stream through your whole being with every breath you take.

Let your mind be at ease as the yellow mist lightens your skin and soothes it.

Imagine that nature is all in harmony with this yellow and you are in harmony with nature. Experience the feeling of freedom you make in your head.

Then imagine a silky yellow ribbon, softly flowing around you, wrapping the mist of harmony and consciousness around your body with a blanket of soft, calming tranquility, as we did before.

Breathe in the velvety yellow mist as it bathes you in a calm ocean, taking all the space you need to feel deep relaxation.

Step Five: Then imagine you're floating on a green mist, actually start seeing, hearing, imagining and experiencing a green mist all around you, absorbing your hair, feeling submerged in the green mist, a beautiful green color. Green grass-like lush.

And as you breathe in this warm, green mist, the gentle softness is all around your heart and you sense that your heart is starting to relax all around that area, all the way up to your throat area. Imagine you can feel your heart expanding, opening and connecting to the world around you as you relax.

Imagine your chest and heart area now vibrating to the green color and enjoying the peace and relaxation it brings. Start feeling this green bringing comfort across your body, gentle softness, this beautiful green color.

The green absorbs everything unwanted around your soul, floats it away, takes it away, leaving in its place only harmony, balance and comfort. If you breathe in the green mist, visualize and feel your body becoming even limper, looser, stronger and more relaxed.

Experience the green purification and liberating you, allowing your body to function in perfect harmony with nature as planned. Then imagine a green ribbon smooth, silky, flowing around you... Like the previous measure.

Step Six: Well, just imagine floating on a blue mist now. Only invest your mind in the idea that on this beautiful blue color you float smoothly. Allow your throat and neck to relax up through the back of your neck to feel calm and relaxed with your throat and neck. Breathe in the blue air and feel it all over your body moving and floating. Enable all the muscles in your body to draw up and soften and balance this gentle blue water. Think your body is at ease as it functions and soothes the blue fog.

Imagine carrying something unwanted with the blue mist, leaving only comfort, ease, and protection.

Imagine once again that all creation is in harmony with blue and that you are in harmony with nature. The body has been beautifully designed to work in harmony with nature, so let all the natural processes of just' being' happen to you as you do this.

Feel the warmth rising inside you as the blue mist fills every cell and muscle and now imagine the silky ribbon flowing around your body, covering your skin softly with a blue mist blanket, soaking you in a sea of complete relaxation.

Step 7: Then imagine yourself floating on a misty violet cloud, a beautiful violet-rosy shade, a very gentle combination that produces beautiful lavender color.

Imagine that your body is penetrated by the soft color of a violet, that very soft purple, and let yourself go deeper into your mind. Imagine drawing this violet in your skin. Experience the beautiful color that gives you peace and serenity.

Make sure that this beautiful soft violet mist makes you feel safe and relaxed. Tune into nature, relax into this natural feeling with the violet color in which you are and start breathing in the soft violet mist. Breathe it in and feel your mind's muscles working in harmony with nature's intent.

Feel relaxed, feel the wonderful things happening right now within your body.

Step Eight: Imagine now within your mind a mixture of all the colors you've been dreaming about creating a rainbow and surrounding you throughout this technique. Imagine merging them to create a beautiful white light that purifies, cleanses, fills the body and mind with the glorious sense of comfort, rejuvenation, and balance.

Right at the top of your head, bring the light in, a beautiful clear bright light, flowing down your whole body, filling all the gaps between all the cells, giving you the comfort of knowing that you deserve the experience of a happy, healthy, energetic existence.

Step Nine: Now let yourself be immersed in this beautiful rainbow of life's energy, let your mind and body be very responsive, open to creating the experience you want and deserve.

Bask for as long as you like in the colors.

Step Ten: You should encourage yourself to return to the consciousness of the position you're in when you're ready. Explain to yourself that you feel very good, very balanced and energized when you open your eyes. Then open your eyes, wiggle your fingers and toes, relax and enjoy being more relaxed and refreshed.

CHAPTER NINE:
Exploring Yoga In Chakra System

T The chakra system is basically a system of energy hubs across the spinal column, each acting as a focal point of psychophysical energy transmission and reception. Ironically, as the position of the chakras overlaps with that of the glands, there seems to be a strong relationship between the chakras and the neuroendocrine system. The glands are responsible for directly secreting hormones into the bloodstream, establishing the body's chemical balance. The chakras are situated along the spinal column and each of the energy centers specializes in a different aspect of our perceptions of body, mind, and spirit that leads to the aura that we are bringing through the universe.

The system's lower chakras are the most dominant since they reflect our animal instincts like survival, sexuality, and supremacy. The upper chakras enter a more spiritual level when you climb the energy column. To balance, the life of the Self (I am-ness), the upper and lower chakras must be aligned. When the Self emanates from the midpoint of the heart chakra to its fullest potential, the quest for spirituality comes from a place of love.

The word "chakra" means "ring," and to those who can see them, they appear to be a kind of spinning wheel of light. By releasing subtle energy into the aura and the part of the physical body where they are located, the chakras transform this light (life force/prana/ chi). Unbalanced chakras can result in physical imbalances. It is, therefore, possible that the ultimate cause of infection could be the disharmonious, unbalanced or inadequate stream of subtle energy through the chakras.

The seven major chakras are Muladhara (root), Svadisthana (sacral), Manipura (navel), Anahata (heart), Vishudda (throat), Ajna (brow) and Sahasrara (crown) from the lowest instinctual chakra to the highest spiritual chakra.

Muladhara (Root / Base) Chakra At the base of the sacrum and the coccyx is the root chakra. It is associated with the earth's dimension and the lower limbs and is related to the adrenal glands energetically. When Muladhara is imbalanced, fear, fighting or flight responses and a sense of being rootless-out of touch with gravity can be formed. On the opposite, by the practice of Asanas (Frog, Bridge, and 1/2 pigeon), by the color red and with the mantra LAM, we can stimulate Muladhara to encourage a good sense of security, positive self-image and groundedness.

Svadisthana (Sacral / Sex) Chakra Svadisthana is located in the center of the navel and pubic bone and is connected with the dimension of water and sexual energy. The relation with the neuroendocrine system seems to be through the sex glands (ovaries/testicles) which stimulate and retain sexual characteristics and behavioral influences. It can result in primitive emotions and lust when Svadisthana is imbalanced. But with a focus on the color orange, the mantra VAM and Asanas (pigeon, cobra, sphinx and half locust) we can build vitality and desire, imagination and sensuality from the sacral chakra energy.

Manipura (Navel / Solar Plexus) Chakra The navel chakra can be located halfway between the sternum base and the navel and is associated with the principle of fire and personal power. It is linked to the pancreas which holds our body's blood sugar levels, which in turn affects our energy levels. With a sense of helplessness, fear of change, feelings of being trapped, and sometimes brute force acts, Manipura or "jewel town" can negatively affect us. Nevertheless, with the mantra RAM and the color yellow and the practice of Bow, Full Locust, and Warrior postures, we can nourish our navel chakra by meditating, we can benefit from the strength, flexibility, calm confidence and adaptability as well as openness to change.

Anahata (Heart) Chakra Find your heart chakra in the center of your sternum as the title describes. Anahata is the chakra system's energetic core and is aligned with the component of water, the cardiovascular system, and others ' compassion. The heart chakra connects through the heart and thymus gland to the glandular system, influencing immunity and love production. Ignoring Anahata may result in a sense of desperation and hardheartedness, but one can develop a Self of empathy and unconditional love for the world through the practice of Camel and Fish postures, the green color and the YAM mantra.

Vishudda (Throat) Chakra Vishudda rests in the throat's hollow and is associated with the ether dimension, the auditory system, self-expression, power, and strength. The relation between the throat chakra and the neuroendocrine system is the thyroid gland which secretes hormones that influence the body's metabolism. Imbalanced, Vishudda could leave you with a perception of the world prejudiced and stiffness to alter. On the other side, stimulating your throat chakra with Shoulder stand and Plow pose and meditating with the blue color and the HAM mantra will spark your sense of reason, reasoning, creative expression and devotion to truth-speaking.

Ajna (Third Eye / Brow) Chakra Go between your eyebrows to find your third eye chakra related to the light dimension, sensory input, intuition, telepathic communication, and meditative capacity. Ajna has a link to the hypophyseal gland which contributes to the nervous system reception and hormone secretions. The imbalanced Ajna would contribute to our desire to control things and our narrow-mindedness by blocking the path to Samadhi. But through the practice of Yoga Mudra and concentration on the color indigo purple and the mantra OM, insight, creative thinking and a wider view of life can nourish our energy system.

Sahasrara (Crown) Chakra You are blossoming your crown chakra at the highest energy center in the chakra system, at the top of your head. Practice sitting in lotus pose in silent meditation to prevent a loss of awareness and feelings of being put down or isolation. Reflect on the function of the pineal gland to establish the ability to see inside-pure intuitive perception. Concentrate your imagination on a violet white lotus blossom that opens up at your head's crown and absorbs the fragrance of celestial knowledge and harmony with everything that comes to you.

The Centre of Our Existence!

Most of us have heard or read about the seven energy centers that we call Chakras. We assume that these are very essential centers of our being in terms of our energy field, our aura, and most of all our equilibrium which can manifest in our physical body.

So what can we do about these energies and how can these centers be balanced? You don't need a high schooling degree, but maybe just a few little tips that can improve your interaction with these chakras ' different levels.

Generally, these chakras are aligned with colors. Not just to differentiate or classify them from each other, but because our emotional psychology is powered by colors on their own. Instead of seven, they deal with nine chakras individually. We're going to go through the nine chakras and describe their characteristics.

The characteristics of the Chakras are described as follows, having worked with them through my meditation and healing for many years: we will start from the bottom up.

The Root Chakra is the first chakra at the base of the spine, it is color being "gold" and its secondary color being "black." Its features are rooted in a body to the life of the earth system. It holds stability, protection, and survival of basic needs. Central body parts of the Chakra include the arms, thighs, rectum, lungs, ribs, stomach, and lower back in our body. This Chakra will be healed and balanced by any red or black gemstones. Preferred gemstones: Garnet, red ruby, smoky quartz, and black obsidian.

The Belly Chakra is the second Chakra in the belly, the shade of which is "Red." Their characteristics are our individuality, self-esteem, self-power, and world power. This Chakra accesses the psychological body's lower level and houses the unhealed inner child of one. Here is where the memories of this life, as well as past-life traumas, are kept. This Chakra is based on the ability to let go of old emotions. This chakra is very heavy. Belly Chakra body parts of our body include ovaries, breasts, penis, uterus, lumbar spine, kidneys, bladder, and broad bowel. This Chakra will cure and balance any orange gemstones. Preferred gemstones: carnelian (pregnancy assistance) and coral.

The Solar Plexus Chakra is the third chakra in the stomach with a "Yellow" hue. The conscious and logical mind is its characteristics. There is a representation of our personal power, intuition and self-confidence,. The emphasis here is on business, mathematical meaning, and material learning capacity, as well as our self-empowerment and will. The inner child is held there as part of the heart, and that can help bring us our tools for survival. The body parts of Solar Plexus include the heart, uterus, pancreas, small intestine, liver, and gall bladder. This Chakra will cure and balance any yellow gemstones. Preferred gemstones: Sapphire Citrine and Orange.

The Heart Chakra is the fourth Chakra in the heart and its color is either "blue" or "pink" in the persona state of mind as a secondary color. Pink is going to represent earthly love and seek love for the man. Green as a symbol of empathy is the more basic and unconditional love for self and humanity. The characteristics are that giving and receiving love is very significant. It's about being able to love yourself and others. Body parts of the heart chakra are the chest, circulatory system, lungs, shoulder, and upper back. This Chakra can cure and balance every color of pink or green gemstones. Recommended gemstones: for the Green Malachite and Modalvite, and the Kunzite and Pink Crystal Quartz.

The Throat Chakra is the fifth Chakra in the throat, with the "Dark Blue" color. The characteristics are speech, hearing (including mental hearing), receiving others, interaction, and imagination. This comprises the human body's blueprint. Possibility of change, rebirth, and healing are found here, including by karmic release healing one's potential verses of the past. The frustration can be held by the throat and what we need to let go of. The body parts of the throat chakra include the chest, head, chin, teeth, ears, eyes, and thyroid gland. This Chakra is healed and balanced by light blue gemstones. Suggest gemstones: Aquamarine, Turkish and Blue Tourmaline.

The Chakra of the Third Eye is the sixth Chakra in our brows and its shade is "Indigo." The features are where we see to grasp the non-physical reality beyond physical realities into the mental world. It's known as Goddess Within's location. The body parts of the Third Eye Chakra include the ears, mouth, and brain. This Chakra is healed and balanced by any indigo gemstones. Preferred gemstones: Sapphire and Azurite.

The Crown Chakra is the seventh Chakra on our body, the color of which is "Violet." The characteristics it is the first point that the soul enters the body at birth by traveling back into this plane. It's known as the Goddess's location. The body parts of the Crown Chakra include the spine and nervous systems. This Chakra will cure and balance any violet gemstones. Preferred gemstones: Serenite and Amethyst.

The Chakra Contact Point, as we name it, is the eighth Chakra found just a few inches from the Chakra crown and its color is "pure or white." This is where contact will take place with your guides and loved ones, bringing clarity to guide and harmony in your connection. It's beyond our physical body and never impacts us. This Chakra is healed and balanced by any white or transparent rock. Preferred gemstones: Clear Quartz and Pink.

Harmony with the Chakra origin, as we call it, is the ninth Chakra, a few feet higher than the Chakra Connection Point, and its color is "Silver." This is the stage the soul is working on. For each of us as individuals, the experience of meditating on this will vary as our soul-level experiences are special to each one of us for our soul-level development. It is a very high and strong chakra, and some people may find this uncomfortable. Using its strength will take some practice. We have never used any Gemstone for this Chakra, but the entire Chakra must be balanced so that it can work properly. To cure and balance it, you can use a combination of the eight Gemstones from the various Chakras.

I usually use the last two chakras, but when you start meditating, they are not required when you first begin to use your chakras. Once you get to know your center points and try to tap into their energies then these Chakras will give you some help and they will have an impact on you.

Chakras are a very important part of our lives and this may or may not be acknowledged. It's an option for yourself. Whatever your preference on the subject is, in your daily life you can feel its influence.

Relaxation of Peace With Elemental Healing

Holy and ancient scriptures talk of the body being formed with 5 natural elements that created the whole universe— Fire, Water, Earth, Sky, and Ether. Those who do not believe in religion but have a spiritual world value, they also claim that we are part of the Paramatma— the ultimate reality and consciousness. Those who are skeptics and believe in science alone are not likely to know what the Big Bang Theory means. This says the entire world consisted of various "Elements" separated by an explosion, and the vibrations created life and arranged the rest of the components. It's a known fact among all religious believers and saints that "God created us in His way," meaning-God being the maker, we are the same; and if He can kill, we can do the same thing. And the whole point of saying that was that we have complete control over our body system; we can naturally create positivity and kill any kind of infection in our body. That simply proves that our body is made up of all the 5 elements listed above. Those who believe in spirituality tell us that we have seven chakras in our body and that each chakra has a component in it.

1. Root Chakra (Muladhara)-it is named the base of life and is made up of the element of Earth. This foundation chakra contains both our spiritual powers and ability. Healing this chakra is very important to maintain a balance in life. If you have issues with your spine, cure your mooladhar chakra. The Earth's heart is believed to be connected to it.

2. Sacral Chakra (Swadhishthaan)-all our animal instincts are known to have this chakra. The sacral chakra drives all of our sexual desires. If you have any womb or fertility problems, cure your swadhishthan chakra. It consists of the dimension of Fire. Lower levels of the component cause the digestive process to slow down, and too much of the digestive process

contributes to excessive irritation due to piled up heat energy.

3. Naval Chakra (Manipur) — the functioning of two vital organs— liver and kidneys and pancreas are all related to the naval chakra. This chakra also consists of the element of Fire. Any other element's intervention contributes to a significant imbalance and causes damage to the liver and kidneys. Ascites-fluid accumulation in the abdominal cavity, for instance, suggesting that the liver is afflicted with some major diseases such as cirrhosis, and therefore needs proper treatment. So the water element interferes with the fire element, causing trouble in the body.

4. Heart Chakra (Anaahat) is the core of all our emotions and feelings. This chakra must be full of light as the soul is considered to be in this chakra's location. This regulates the breathing, heart and blood circulation in the body along with our emotions and feelings being controlled. It is the core of love that is unconditional. To lead a happy and healthy life, we need to disable and

heal it. This chakra is known to consist of the component of Air.

5. Throat Chakra (Vishuddhi)-all the saints say that if you can make your vishuddhi chakra powerful, you will have "Vaak Siddhi," that is, whatever you say is true. It's like being a prophet with divine authority to pronounce and decree words that would materialize in the real world. It does a detoxifier's work. The name says it's The Purifier itself. The vishuddhi chakra can annul all the toxic air we breathe in or any toxin in the body. It is said that Lord Shiva, with his vishuddhi Chakra, kept the poison carried from the Sagar Manthan. It also regulates the glands of the salivary and the thyroid gland. You must choose to cure the Vishuddhhi chakra to get rid of any skin disease, thyroid or cancer.

6. Third Eye Chakra (Aagya Chakra)-It is the source of all the conscious, sub-conscious perceptions of old and unconscious days. The third-eye chakra gives us a strong memory, builds spatial awareness, and gives us control over our lives. Our consciousness becomes very

aware when it is triggered correctly and then it actively directs us into what to do, where to go, who to obey, etc. This provides us with insight and regulates our processes of visual, nasal (Olfactory) and hearing. This chakra consists of the component of Ether, which is Space.

7. Crown Chakra (Sahasrara)— the most powerful of all is the pituitary gland Sahasrara chakra— the master gland. We get to feel the Supreme Conscious when it is triggered. This regulates all the functions of the body as it controls the brain that is the whole body's command processing system. When this chakra is packed with the right amount of energy, we obtain Enlightenment. It is made up of the component of the Ether.

These are some of the religious truths that can be of great benefit to our body's relaxation and healing. We are said to have an etheric body and a physical body. Our spiritual body is the etheric body that is directly proportionate to our physical health. Because we can't all meditate for long hours every day, having some therapeutic spa facilities such as aromatherapy and

Asian Body Massages would be the most viable solution to our recovery.

Aromatherapy stimulates all senses and automatically strengthens the chakras. Asian massages are very effective because with acupressure methods the oils they use and the strokes that are used are applied. Panchkarma is a naturopathic therapy in which they offer body massages of various types, acupressure, Shirodhara, steam baths, and a strictly regulated diet. It would motivate you to have a balanced mind and body by visiting any of the best spas around you. Spiritual science says that we can not cure ourselves of any disease. All we need to do is have harmony in all our body components that can be accomplished by Elemental Healing and Chakra Healing. Once you are in the care of professional masseurs who know exactly how to energize your body, you will enter a happy and peaceful state. Relaxation, Divine Recovery, and Peace— all three things happen at the same time, with only the right choice.

Chakras: The soul of Energy Medicine

Originating in ancient India and China, Eastern philosophy and medicine have historically viewed body structures and life processes as inseparable within them. Ancient language remains halfway between structure and function and describes other forces in the human body, describing the flow of life energy and conduits for that flow that do not conform with Western science and medicine accepted anatomical structures. The chakras are the energy centers in the biological field of an individual and are responsible for their physiological and psychological state as well as for certain organs classes. The power that spins in the chakras influences all the vital functions of the human body. These can be described as "referred to as whirlpools," and in Indian they are referred to as "energy bursts" or "wheels." Exactly in these centers, the process of energy conversion takes place. Vital energy circulates in the chakras along with blood around the meridians, supplying all organs and processes in the human body. The human body is vulnerable to various disorders when the movement in these meridians stagnates. Chi

Gun, an ancient Chinese self-healing system that triggers the energy centers, is an excellent preventive tool specifically designed to combat such stagnation. Through massaging specific areas corresponding to the various chakras, Chi Gun teaches people to release the power themselves.

In the Vedic Canons, there are 49 chakras, of which seven are basic; 21 are in the second circle, and 21 are in the fourth. According to the Vedis, there are several streams of energy leading from the chakras to different locations. Three of these are simple outlets. The first, named "Sushumna," is hollow and in the spine is concentrated. On either side of the backbone are the other two energy channels, "ida" and "Pingala." In most citizens, these two channels are the most involved, while "Sushumna" stagnates.

In the body of healthy individuals, the seven essential the high speed of chakras spin and its slowdown in periods of illness or advancing age. The chakras remain partially open when a body was in a harmonious state.

Closed chakras can not obtain power, resulting in different disorders.

"Muladhara," the first essential chakra, is found in the tailbone region at the base of the spine. Life energy is stored in this chakra, which is at the center of a strong and healthy immune system. Without consuming one's reserves of this vital energy, a person can't become sick, old or even die. Muladhara governs the very will to live. It is also responsible for bones and joints, teeth, nails, urinogenital and large intestines. The first signs of a dysfunctional Muladhara are unreasonable fear, fatigue, lack of future security or confidence, issues with the legs and feet, and intestinal disorders.

The Muladhara chakra's disrupted operation triggers food deficiencies, digestive problems, bone and spine diseases, and nervous stress among others.

The second chakra, "Svadhistana," is three or four fingers below the belly button at the bottom of the sacrum. The pelvis, kidneys and sexual functions are regulated by this chakra. Through this chakra, we also sense the feelings of other peoples. Symptoms of a "Svadhistana" failure are liver, cystitis, and arthritis.

In the solar plexus region, the third chakra, "Manipura," is located. This chakra is the core of digestion and breathing energy storage and transmission. It is responsible for hearing, gastrointestinal system, liver, gall bladder, pancreas, and nervous system. Symptoms of stagnant "Manipura" are as follows: intensified and persistent worrying disorders as well as disorders of the heart, liver, and nerve.

In the chest area is the fourth chakra, "Anahata," also called the heart chakra. Through this chakra, we produce and perceive love. It is responsible for the chest, the lungs, the bronchi, the arms, and hands. Depression and cardiac imbalances are signs of stagnation.

The fifth chakra, "Vishudha," is the core for analytical skills and reasoning at the throat level. This chakra, along with the trachea and lungs, protects the body, hearing organs. Symptoms include a lack of emotional control, cervical spine pain, sore throats, communication difficulties, and ailments of the esophagus and thyroid.

The sixth chakra, "Adjna," is found between the brows of the eye and is considered the "fifth eye." "Adjna" circulates energy to the head and hypophysis and is also responsible for determining our harmonious growth. If the "third eye" of a person ceases the functioning properly, a fall in intellectual ability, migraines and headaches, olfactory diseases, , earaches and psychological disorders may be observed.

"Sahasrara," the seventh chakra, is located at the very top of the head and represents the apex where the power of an individual vibrates at the highest frequency. It is known as a religious hub of cosmic energy and the entrance to the soul. A stagnant "Sahasrara," as well as a lack of basic intuition, may result in a decrease in or loss of inner wisdom.

With this basic knowledge of the first seven chakras, we may address the question: "How do we use this information to identify the causes of our troubles and problems and learn to control the functions of the chakras ourselves with the aid of Eastern Medicine?."

From Eastern Medicine's viewpoint, our wellbeing depends on the distribution of our knowledge area of energy-consciousness. A power deficit inevitably causes anxiety. The only difference between youth and old age and between a sick and healthy adult, according to Tibetan Medicine, is the difference in the rotational speed of the chakras ' whirlpool energy centers. If these multiple speeds are regulated, the aged will rejuvenate and the sick will recover. Therefore, restoring and sustaining a healthy flow of energy centers is the best way to preserve and sustain our wellbeing, youth, and vitality.

A collection of physical exercises is the best way to keep the chakras healthy. Yannis did not just name them drills, but routines. Such rituals allow the human body to shape to an ideal level of function its energy centers. Each morning and in the evening, if not necessary, the seven rituals, one for each chakra, must be performed together. Skipping habits unbalances the distribution of power, so you should skip no more than one day a week for the best results. The regular chakra rituals are required not only to revitalize the body but also to make every facet of life effective. "You'll also become happier when you know how to convert your power," Yannis concluded.

To know these practices (which have changed the lives of many peoples throughout the world), it is much more important to see them in action than to try to follow written explanations or maps. A DVD, available from Helix 7, Inc. (www. FeelingOfHappiness.com), contains actual ritual presentations.

Meditation is another way to keep the chakras balanced and in their optimum half-open state. Meditative approaches are fundamental to human experience; they have accrued through many different cultures over the years and have shown their importance in achieving peace, insight, equanimity and transcendent desperation. People who regularly meditate are typically calmer, healthier, happier, and more productive people. During their daily lives, they are more successful as they make full use of their mental and physical capacity, talents and skill. Often, Humans fail to realize theat great dormant forces that in the bodies are still unawakened. We need to know how to recycle and use them. Only mindfulness can achieve this. More than 1000 years ago, Eastern men of knowledge, who believed that meditation was a critical necessity, came upon this discovery. With the strength of their minds, they learned to manipulate their internal organs and regulate their metabolism. For the brain, meditation is what exercise is for the body; it can build up mental strength just like physical strength. Just as it is important for an individual to train his or her body in sports, meditation is important for an individual to train their minds.

Early morning is the best time for meditation, ideally at midnight. Do not meditate when you are sad, angry, anxious or ill, because these constant disturbances of emotion and physiology make a calm state of mind difficult. It is best to arrange the undistracted solitude of a peaceful, clean room with flowers or Mother Nature's calming sounds-near a lake, river, waterfall, forest or fields-for an active meditation session.

CONCLUSION

A river of pulsating white healing energy begins to flow out and down the body's left side from the Crown chakra. It's about 3 "long. It's vibrating and pulsating. This 3" ribbon flows down the face's left side. Your back, shoulder, left arm, butt, thigh, knee, leg down to your left ankle. Then this 3 "rope of healing white light passes under your foot and up the right ankle. Then the right leg, hip, knee, arm, back, neck side of the head and into the crown chakra. You have a 3" circle of white healing, pulsating, complex healing white light circling the body from left to right. From your crown chakra under your feet and back to the chakra of the crown.

Now the second circle of power to heal. A 2 "rope of white healing light starts from your Crown chakra and begins to flow down your body's forehead. Down your forehead, your face, your nose, your lips, your mouth, your arms, your heart, your belly, your groin, your thighs, your knees, your legs down to your feet. Then the back of your arms, knees, buttocks, to the base of your coccyx spine, to the neck, and the Crown chakra, to the medulla oblongata. You now have around your body two strong circles. One from left to right, one from back to front. Sit there and bask in the energy of the middle pillar with the 5 shinings, pulsating spheres and the 3 "pipe down the center. Then feel the energy of the 2 rings as they rotate around your body from front to back and from left to right. Now from the ground chakra, a 3" white healing light rope starts to curl around your ankles. It's like a bandage of ases and starts to cover you like a bandage of mummies. Your feet, thighs, buttocks, and genitals are wrapped in the 3 "ribbon. The lower back, back, chest, arms, shoulders, neck, face and head and into the chakra of the Crown. You are tightly wrapped in a 3" ribbon of strong, pulsating, white light. You have your middle pillar of 5 circles, your 3 "line down the center of your body, a circle running from left to right around your body and a ring going from front to back. Now a full energy cover. Stop for a minute and experience this pulsating, powerful white light energy streaming around the outside and inside your body.

www.ingramcontent.com/pod-product-compliance
Lightning Source LLC
Chambersburg PA
CBHW061343250726
48657CB00004B/1306